JIMD Reports
Volume 39

Eva Morava
Editor-in-Chief

Matthias Baumgartner · Marc Patterson ·
Shamima Rahman · Johannes Zschocke
Editors

Verena Peters
Managing Editor

JIMD Reports
Volume 39

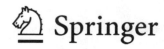 Springer

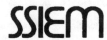

Editor-in-Chief
Eva Morava
Tulane University Medical School
New Orleans
Louisiana
USA

Editor
Matthias Baumgartner
Division of Metabolism & Children's Research
Centre
University Children's Hospital Zürich
Zürich
Switzerland

Editor
Marc Patterson
Division of Child and Adolescent Neurology
Mayo Clinic
Rochester
Minnesota
USA

Editor
Shamima Rahman
Clinical and Molecular Genetics Unit
UCL Institute of Child Health
London
UK

Editor
Johannes Zschocke
Division of Human Genetics
Medical University Innsbruck
Innsbruck
Austria

Managing Editor
Verena Peters
Center for Child and Adolescent Medicine
Heidelberg University Hospital
Heidelberg
Germany

ISSN 2192-8304   ISSN 2192-8312   (electronic)
JIMD Reports
ISBN 978-3-662-57576-5   ISBN 978-3-662-57577-2   (eBook)
https://doi.org/10.1007/978-3-662-57577-2

Contents

Successful Pregnancy in a Young Woman with Multiple Acyl-CoA Dehydrogenase Deficiency   1
Annalisa Creanza, Mariella Cotugno, Cristina Mazzaccara, Giulia Frisso,
Giancarlo Parenti, and Brunella Capaldo

Role of Intramuscular Levofolinate Administration in the Treatment of Hereditary Folate Malabsorption: Report of Three Cases   7
Emanuela Manea, Paul Gissen, Simon Pope, Simon J. Heales, and Spyros Batzios

The Prevalence of PMM2-CDG in Estonia Based on Population Carrier Frequencies and Diagnosed Patients   13
Mari-Anne Vals, Sander Pajusalu, Mart Kals, Reedik Mägi, and Katrin Õunap

Triheptanoin: A Rescue Therapy for Cardiogenic Shock in Carnitine-acylcarnitine Translocase Deficiency   19
Sidharth Mahapatra, Amitha Ananth, Nancy Baugh, Mihaela Damian,
and Gregory M. Enns

Glutaric Aciduria Type 1 and Acute Renal Failure: Case Report and Suggested Pathomechanisms   25
Marcel du Moulin, Bastian Thies, Martin Blohm, Jun Oh, Markus J. Kemper,
René Santer, and Chris Mühlhausen

Cardiovascular Histopathology of a 11-Year Old with Mucopolysaccharidosis VII Demonstrates Fibrosis, Macrophage Infiltration, and Arterial Luminal Stenosis   31
Valerie Lew, Louis Pena, Robert Edwards, and Raymond Y. Wang

Longitudinal Changes in White Matter Fractional Anisotropy in Adult-Onset Niemann-Pick Disease Type C Patients Treated with Miglustat   39
Elizabeth A. Bowman, Dennis Velakoulis, Patricia Desmond,
and Mark Walterfang

Beta-Ketothiolase Deficiency Presenting with Metabolic Stroke After a Normal Newborn Screen in Two Individuals   45
Monica H. Wojcik, Klaas J. Wierenga, Lance H. Rodan, Inderneel Sahai,
Sacha Ferdinandusse, Casie A. Genetti, Meghan C. Towne, Roy W. A. Peake,
Philip M. James, Alan H. Beggs, Catherine A. Brownstein, Gerard T. Berry,
and Pankaj B. Agrawal

Rapidly Progressive White Matter Involvement in Early Childhood:
The Expanding Phenotype of Infantile Onset Pompe?   55
A. Broomfield, J. Fletcher, P. Hensman, R. Wright, H. Prunty, J. Pavaine,
and S.A. Jones

Four Years' Experience in the Diagnosis of Very Long-Chain Acyl-CoA
Dehydrogenase Deficiency in Infants Detected in Three Spanish Newborn
Screening Centers   63
B. Merinero, P. Alcaide, E. Martín-Hernández, A. Morais, M. T. García-Silva,
P. Quijada-Fraile, C. Pedrón-Giner, E. Dulin, R. Yahyaoui, J. M. Egea,
A. Belanger-Quintana, J. Blasco-Alonso, M. L. Fernandez Ruano, B. Besga,
I. Ferrer-López, F. Leal, M. Ugarte, P. Ruiz-Sala, B. Pérez, and C. Pérez-Cerdá

Social Functioning and Behaviour in Mucopolysaccharidosis IH
[Hurlers Syndrome]   75
Annukka Lehtonen, Stewart Rust, Simon Jones, Richard Brown,
and Dougal Hare

Mitochondrial Encephalopathy and Transient 3-Methylglutaconic Aciduria
in ECHS1 Deficiency: Long-Term Follow-Up   83
Irene C. Huffnagel, Egbert J. W. Redeker, Liesbeth Reneman, Frédéric M. Vaz,
Sacha Ferdinandusse, and Bwee Tien Poll-The

Glutaric Aciduria Type 3: Three Unrelated Canadian Cases, with Different
Routes of Ascertainment   89
Paula J. Waters, Thomas M. Kitzler, Annette Feigenbaum, Michael T. Geraghty,
Osama Al-Dirbashi, Patrick Bherer, Christiane Auray-Blais, Serge Gravel,
Nathan McIntosh, Komudi Siriwardena, Yannis Trakadis,
Catherine Brunel-Guitton, and Walla Al-Hertani

High-Throughput Screen Fails to Identify Compounds That Enhance
Residual Enzyme Activity of Mutant N-Acetyl-α-Glucosaminidase
in Mucopolysaccharidosis Type IIIB   97
O. L. M. Meijer, P. van den Biggelaar, R. Ofman, F. A. Wijburg,
and N. van Vlies

Demographic and Psychosocial Influences on Treatment Adherence
for Children and Adolescents with PKU: A Systematic Review 107
Emma Medford, Dougal Julian Hare, and Anja Wittkowski

JIMD Reports
DOI 10.1007/8904_2017_38

RESEARCH REPORT

Successful Pregnancy in a Young Woman with Multiple Acyl-CoA Dehydrogenase Deficiency

Annalisa Creanza · Mariella Cotugno ·
Cristina Mazzaccara · Giulia Frisso ·
Giancarlo Parenti · Brunella Capaldo

Received: 07 March 2017 / Revised: 08 June 2017 / Accepted: 09 June 2017 / Published online: 07 July 2017
© SSIEM and Springer-Verlag Berlin Heidelberg 2017

Abstract Multiple acyl-CoA dehydrogenation deficiency (MADD) is an inborn disorder of fatty acid oxidation due to a defect *in electron transfer to the respiratory chain*. We describe the medical/nutritional management of a successful pregnancy in a 19-year-old woman with a known diagnosis of MADD. A high-carbohydrate, low-fat, six-meal diet supplemented with protein was prescribed to meet the nutritional needs during pregnancy. L-Carnitine supplementation was also progressively increased over the weeks. Serum acyl-carnitine profile revealed raised levels of chain-length C6-C14, which remained substantially unchanged during pregnancy. Serum amino acid profile was in the normal range indicating an adequate nutritional support. Pregnancy progressed uneventful and the patient gave birth to a healthy boy without any complication.

A careful clinical monitoring associated with an adequate medical/nutritional management may improve pregnancy outcome in women with MADD.

Communicated by: Robert Steiner

A. Creanza · M. Cotugno · B. Capaldo (✉)
Department of Clinical Medicine and Surgery, University of Naples
Federico II, Naples, Italy
e-mail: bcapaldo@unina.it

C. Mazzaccara · G. Frisso
Department of Molecular Medicine and Biotechnologies, CEINGE-
Biotecnologie Avanzate, University of Naples Federico II, Naples,
Italy

G. Parenti
Department of Translational Medicine (G.P.), University of Naples
Federico II, Naples, Italy

Introduction

Multiple acyl-CoA dehydrogenase deficiency (MADD), also known as glutaric aciduria type II, is an autosomal recessively inherited disease of fatty acid, some amino acid and choline oxidation, caused by a defect in the electron transfer flavoprotein (ETF) or the electron transfer flavoprotein dehydrogenase (ETFDH), enzymes involved in the mitochondrial respiratory chain. This defect results in compromised fatty acid oxidation, with consequent impaired adenosine triphosphate (ATP) synthesis, insufficient gluconeogenesis and excessive lipid accumulation in different organs.

The clinical expression of MADD is highly heterogeneous ranging from severe neonatal-onset form, with or without congenital anomalies, to milder form with a late-onset, which is characterized by intermittent episodes of lethargy, metabolic acidosis, non-ketotic hypoglycaemia, muscle weakness, generally triggered by catabolic stress (Rhead et al. 1987; Turnbull et al. 1988; Mongini et al. 1992).

The clinical diagnosis of MADD is based on the presence of organic acid and acylglycine derivatives in the urine and increased levels of medium- and long-chain acyl-carnitines in the blood. Mutations in *ETFA*, *ETFB* or *ETFDH* genes, encoding the alpha and beta subunits of electron transfer flavoprotein and the ETF-dehydrogenase, confirm the diagnosis.

The treatment of MADD consists of a high-carbohydrate, low-fat, low-protein diet associated with riboflavin and carnitine supplementation. Prevention of fasting and of other precipitating stresses is also essential. Riboflavin is precursor of flavin adenine dinucleotide (FAD), a cofactor of several mitochondrial enzymes, such as the acyl-CoA dehydrogenases. There is evidence of symptoms restoration after riboflavin treatment particularly in patients with late-onset MADD (Olsen ct al. 2007).

Advances in both nutritional therapy and management of acute attacks have considerably improved the outcome of MADD, particularly in patients with the milder forms of the disease (Williams et al. 2008; Trakadis et al. 2012). Thus, an increasing number of women long to have a baby. For most of the inherited diseases there is a lack of specific guidelines for the management during pregnancy; therefore, experience from isolated case reports is particularly valuable.

We present the case of a young woman with MADD who led to a successful pregnancy and her medical/nutritional management during pregnancy and delivery.

Case Description

The patient is a 19-year-old woman who was diagnosed with MADD at the age of 3 years, due to occurrence of lethargy and asthenia associated with anorexia. Routine biochemical analyses showed remarkable increments in transaminases, lactic dehydrogenase, aldolase and creatine kinase. The chromatographic layout of urinary organic acids showed a typical dicarboxylic aciduria. MADD diagnosis was confirmed by molecular analysis, performed according to the standardized approach (Scolamiero et al. 2015), which showed a compound heterozygosity in the *ETFDH* gene (NM_001281737.1) for the mutations c.1074G>C (p.R358S) and c.1073G>A (p.R358K) in exon 9. Her parents were healthy carriers of one of the two mutations (Fig. 1).

Since the diagnosis, the patient was under follow up at the Paediatric Unit of AOU Federico II of Naples; she has been treated with a diet restricted in fat and protein associated with riboflavin, pyridoxine and carnitine supplementation. Over the years, the patient required sporadic hospitalizations for metabolic decompensations resolved with intravenous dextrose infusion and hydration.

At the age of 18, the patient was hospitalized for a severe episode of rhabdomyolysis (serum creatine kinase level: 69960UI/L), which resolved with intravenous infusion of

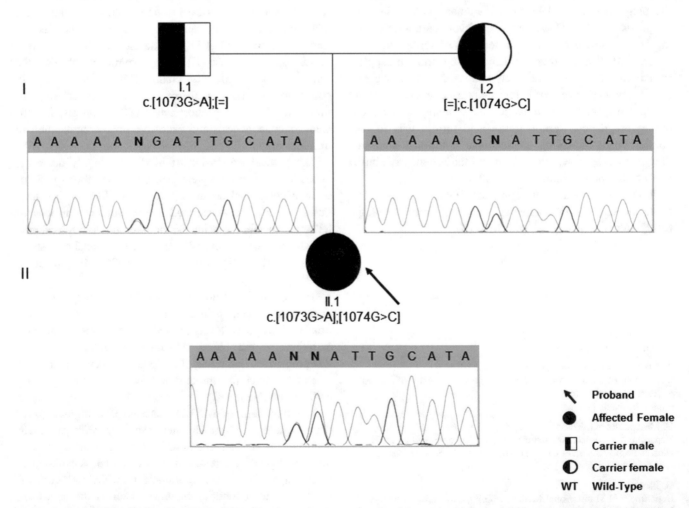

Fig. 1 Pedigrees of the family with MADD defect. The electropherogram showing the mutation in the nucleotide sequence is under each symbol

Dextrose solution (initially 33%, then 10%), hydration and increased oral L-carnitine supplementation (100 mg/kg/day). Few months later, the patient unexpectedly became pregnant. She was not blood related to her partner. The genetic analysis of the partner did not reveal any mutations of *ETFA/ETFB/ETFDH* genes. At 8 week of gestation, the patient was in good clinical conditions and the results of her biochemical routine tests were normal. Echocardiographic examination evidenced a normal cardiac function. The medical and nutritional management for the whole gestation is reported in Table 1. A normocaloric (1,700 kcal) diet moderately restricted in fat and protein was recommended; an adequate intake of carbohydrate (>50% of total calories) was provided since it is the main energy substrate for foetal metabolism. The diet was divided into three main meals and three snacks in order to avoid prolonged fasting and to prevent the risk of hypoglycaemia. In addition, the patient was recommended to have a glucose supply (25–50 g) every 2 h in case of discomfort or episodic vomiting and to contact the hospital in case of persistence of symptoms, fever or acute illness.

In the second and third trimester, a protein supplementation was added to meet the increased protein requirement (Table 1). Riboflavin, pyridoxine and L-carnitine dosages were maintained constant. Folic acid, multivitamin and mineral supplements were started in the first trimester. At the beginning of the third trimester, L-carnitine was increased to 4,000 mg/day because of an increased sense of fatigue.

At the 22nd and the 36th week of pregnancy, the acyl-carnitine profile was analysed through spot extraction of *blood* on filter paper with chromatography liquid-mass tandem spectrometry (LC-MS-MS). *Blood* acyl-carnitine profile revealed raised levels of chain-length C6-C14, which remained substantially stable during pregnancy. *Blood amino acid analysis performed at the same time points showed amino acid levels within or slightly below the normal range* (Table 2).

Periodic glucose home monitoring evidenced blood glucose levels within the normal range and no value was below 70 mg/dL throughout the gestation. Periodic obstetric ultrasound examination evidenced normal foetal growth. At the 39th, the patient underwent an elective cesarean section to reduce the risk of metabolic decompensation. During delivery and in the immediate postoperative period, she received intravenous carnitine (3,000 mg/day) and isotonic solution (with 10% dextrose) at variable rate to maintain normoglycaemia. She gave birth to a 3.1 kg healthy boy without any complication. The baby was breastfed for 2 months during which the patient continued the medical/nutritional therapy followed during pregnancy. At breastfeeding discontinuation, she returned to her usual dietary protein restriction and carnitine was reduced to the pre-gestation dose while continuing riboflavin and pyridoxine.

Discussion

Patients with MADD generate less energy from fatty acids and amino acids because of a defective transfer of electrons from flavoproteins to the mitochondrial respiratory chain. The reduced supply of energy is responsible for a number of clinical manifestations involving particularly those organs that have a high flux of beta-oxidation: the skeletal muscle, with consequent hypotonia, weakness and exercise intolerance; the heart with cardiomyopathy and arrhythmias; the liver with hepatomegaly and liver dysfunction; the brain with encephalopathy.

The severity of the clinical phenotype of MADD is explained by the type of mutation in the *ETFA/ETFB/ETFDH* genes, which results in different levels of residual enzyme activity (Olsen et al. 2003). Nonsense mutations

Table 1 Medical and nutritional management during the course of pregnancy

Week	Weight (kg)	Energy intake (kcal/day)	CHO g (%)	P g (%)	L g (%)	Protein supplement (g/day)	Therapy (mg/day)
8	63.8	1,700	257 (53)	80 (18)	59 (29)	0	L-Carnitine 3,000 Riboflavin 100 Pyridoxine 300
12	65.0	1,900	260 (53)	90 (19)	57 (28)	10	L-Carnitine 3,000 Riboflavin 100 Pyridoxine 300
24	70.0	2,100	263 (49)	110 (21)	60 (30)	30	L-Carnitine 4,000 Riboflavin 100 Pyridoxine 300
34	79.5	2,100	263 (49)	110 (21)	60 (30)	30	L-Carnitine 4,000 Riboflavin 100 Pyridoxine 300

CHO carbohydrate, *P* protein, *L* lipid

Table 2 Blood acyl-carnitine and amino acid profiles during the course of pregnancy

Blood acyl-carnitine levels (μmol/L)				Blood amino acid levels (μmol/L)			
Metabolite	Week 22	Week 36	Normal range	Metabolite	Week 22	Week 36	Normal range
C2	5	4.9	3.5–15.4	Aspartic acid	15	94	24–102
C3	0.28	0.32	0.07–0.65	Glutamic acid	73	298	67–223
C4	0.76	0.35	0.12–0.42	Serine	73	232	111–297
C5	1.35	0.65	0.05–0.24	Glutamine	429	401	432–871
C6	1.12	1.00	0.04–0.18	Alanine	298	554	193–597
C8	3.67	2.74	0.07–0.25	Glycine	145	401	240–460
C10	5.38	5.49	0.09–0.43	Threonine	133	195	109–268
C12	1.21	1.32	0.04–0.21	Arginine	23	76	36–172
C14	0.56	0.53	0.03–0.23	Histidine	87	119	72–131
C16	0.40	0.32	0.01–0.23	Taurine	78	212	50–270
C18	0.19	0.15	0.01–0.18	Tyrosine	46	69	45–107
				Phenylalanine	*62*	*163*	*59–112*
				Methionine	21	32	21–44
				Leucine	98	144	82–258
				Valine	190	237	187–411
				Isoleucine	57	62	42–111
				Lysine	147	195	150–286
				Proline	168	191	50–350
				Ornithine	46	75	63–133

are associated with fatal disease while missense mutations, particularly in the *ETFDH* gene, leaving a detectable residual enzyme activity, may account for the milder forms of the disease (Olsen et al. 2003; Goodman et al. 2002; Schiff et al. 2006; Yotsumoto et al. 2008). In the latter forms, symptoms are usually elicited by illness or catabolic stress, as physical exercise, prolonged fasting, irregular diet, although additional factors, not yet identified, such as cellular temperature, have been reported to modulate the enzymatic activity (Olsen et al. 2003).

Our patient had biallelic mutations in *ETFDH* gene, both in exon 9: c.1074G>C (p.R358S) and c.1073G>A (p. R358K). The former, already described in the homozygous state in three Palestinian siblings, was associated with early onset and milder forms of MADD (Olsen et al. 2005). The c.1073G>A (p.R358K) mutation was submitted just once to ClinVar database (rs796051959 in https://www.ncbi.nlm. nih.gov/clinvar/) as pathogenic allele, although lacking link to a specific clinical condition. However, familial segregation study and in silico analysis, performed by bioinformatics tools, confirmed that this substitution is likely pathogenetic.

Although the mutation identified in our patient cannot be linked with certainty to mild/late-onset MADD, she is likely to have a mild form of the disease in consideration of some important characteristics, i.e., the absence of congenital abnormalities, age at diagnosis and the relatively mild clinical course of the disease. Throughout the years, the patient suffered from sporadic episodes of vomiting, hypoglycaemia and muscle weakness, which were triggered by catabolic stress. Although pregnancy cannot be considered a strictly catabolic condition, it may precipitate metabolic decompensation in women with inherited disorders of energy metabolism. Nausea, recurrent vomiting or fasting may cause a shift of maternal metabolism towards ketosis and reduce glucose availability at a time of increased metabolic demand. Thus, the gestation in a woman with MADD may represent a high-risk condition both for the mother's health and for foetal growth. Hence, strict nutritional/medical surveillance is of paramount importance in pregnant women with MADD. At present, no guidelines are available for the care of pregnant women with this condition. Likewise, a clear management plan for delivery is warranted, as labour is associated with increased energy requirements in addition to fasting and dehydration (Murphy 2015).

In the literature, there is only one case report on pregnancy and delivery in women with MADD (Trakadis et al. 2012). This case refers to a successful pregnancy in a young woman with an atypical presentation of MADD; indeed, no detail of the nutritional management is provided. We planned a close nutritional follow up throughout pregnancy. A six-meal diet high in fibre, very low in fat, but supplemented with protein (10 g/day in the 2nd trimester and 30 g/day in 3rd trimester) was prescribed to meet the increased protein demand during pregnancy. Serum amino acid analysis showed that the amino acid availability was adequate for foetal growth (Elango and Ball 2016). Serum acyl-carnitine concentrations remained stable throughout pregnancy through adequate nutritional therapy along with carnitine, riboflavin and pyridoxine supplements.

The clinical and biochemical stability preserved by the patient during pregnancy demonstrates the safety of the nutritional/medical therapy adopted, which proved to guarantee a good outcome for both mother and baby.

Acknowledgments We thank Dr. Angela Giacco for nutritional counseling.

Synopsis

A successful pregnancy was achieved in a woman with MADD through a careful clinical monitoring associated with an adequate nutritional/medical management.

Authorship Contribution

Annalisa Creanza analysed the data and wrote the first draft, Mariella Cotugno cared for the patient and collected the clinical data, Giulia Frisso and Cristina Mazzaccara performed the genetic test and wrote the part of the manuscript dealing with molecular diagnosis, Giancarlo Parenti cared for the patient during childhood and Brunella Capaldo cared for the patient and revised the manuscript.

Corresponding Author

Brunella Capaldo.

Funding

None.

Compliance with Ethics Guidelines

Conflict of Interest

Annalisa Creanza, Mariella Cotugno, Cristina Mazzaccara, Giulia Frisso, Giancarlo Parenti and Brunella Capaldo declare that they have no conflict of interest.

Informed Consent

All procedures followed were in accordance with the ethical standards of the responsible committee on human experimentation (institutional and national) and with the Helsinki Declaration of 1975, as revised in 2000. Informed consent was obtained from patient for being included in the study. Additional informed consent was obtained from all patients for which identifying information is included in this article.

Animal Rights

This article does not contain any studies with human or animal subjects performed by the any of the authors.

References

Elango R, Ball RO (2016) Protein and amino acid requirements during pregnancy. Adv Nutr 7:839S–844S

Goodman SI, Binard RJ, Woontner MR, Frerman FE (2002) Glutaric acidemia type II: gene structure and mutations of the electron transfer flavoprotein:ubiquinone oxido reductase (ETF:QO) gene. Mol Genet Metab 77:86–90

Mongini T, Doriguzi C, Palmucci L et al (1992) Lipid storage myopathy in multiple acyl-CoA dehydrogenase deficiency: an adult case. Eur Neurol 32:170–176

Murphy E (2015) Pregnancy in women with inherited metabolic disease. Obstet Med 8:61–67

Olsen RK, Andresen BS, Christensen E, Bross P, Skovby F, Gregersen N (2003) Clear relationship between ETF/ETFDH genotype and phenotype in patients with multiple acyl-CoA dehydrogenation deficiency. Hum Mutat 22:12–23

Olsen RK, Andresen BS, Christensen E et al (2005) DNA-based prenatal diagnosis for severe and variant forms of multiple acyl-CoA dehydrogenation deficiency. Prenat Diagn 25:60–64

Olsen RK, Olpin SE, Andresen BS et al (2007) ETFDH mutations as a major cause of riboflavin-responsive multiple acyl-CoA dehydrogenation deficiency. Brain 130:2045–2054

Rhead WJ, Wolff JA, Lipson M et al (1987) Clinical and biochemical variation and family studies in the multiple acyl-CoA dehydrogenation disorders. Pediatr Res 21:371–376

Schiff M, Froissart R, Olsen RK, Acquaviva C, Vianey-Saban C (2006) A novel gross deletion caused by non-homologous recombination of the PDHX gene in a patient with pyruvate dehydrogenase deficiency. Mol Genet Metab 88:153–158

Scolamiero E, Cozzolino C, Albano L et al (2015) Targeted metabolomics in the expanded newborn screening for inborn errors of metabolism. Mol BioSyst 11:1525–1535

Trakadis Y, Kadlubowska D, Barnes R et al (2012) Pregnancy of a patient with multiple Acyl-CoA dehydrogenation deficiency (MADD). Mol Genet Metab 106:491–494

Turnbull DM, Barlett K, Eyre JA et al (1988) Lipid storage myopathy due to glutaric aciduria type II: treatment of a potentially fatal myopathy. Dev Med Child Neurol 30:667–672

Williams SF, Alvarez JR, Pedro HF et al (2008) Glutaric aciduria type II and narcolepsy in pregnancy. Obstet Gynecol 111:522–524

Yotsumoto Y, Hasegawa Y, Fukuda S et al (2008) Clinical and molecular investigations of Japanese cases of glutaric acidemia type 2. Mol Genet Metab 94:61–67

JIMD Reports
DOI 10.1007/8904_2017_39

RESEARCH REPORT

Role of Intramuscular Levofolinate Administration in the Treatment of Hereditary Folate Malabsorption: Report of Three Cases

Emanuela Manea · Paul Gissen · Simon Pope · Simon J. Heales · Spyros Batzios

Received: 31 March 2017 / Revised: 17 May 2017 / Accepted: 09 June 2017 / Published online: 07 July 2017
© SSIEM and Springer-Verlag Berlin Heidelberg 2017

Abstract Hereditary folate malabsorption is a rare autosomal recessive disorder caused by impaired active folate transport across membranes and into the central nervous system due to loss-of-function mutations in proton-coupled folate transporter (PCFT). Newborns with this condition have initially normal folate stores, but as they are unable to absorb dietary folate and use rapidly their stores because of their growth demands, symptoms appear in the early infancy. Significant neurological morbidity usually follows the initial non-specific clinical presentation and delayed initiation of treatment. High dose oral and parenteral folinic acid treatment have been previously reported in literature to improve the clinical outcome without achieving optimal cerebrospinal fluid (CSF) folate levels though. The active isomer of 5-formyltetrahydrofolate, also known as levofolinic acid, is available for administration. We report our experience in achieving normal (age dependent) CSF 5-Methyltetrahydrofolate (5-MTHF) levels following daily intramuscular administration of levofolinic acid in three patients with HFM. Follow-up assessment with repeated lumbar punctures has shown a stabilization of 5-MTHF levels within normal range. Clinical features and brain MRI findings had as well either improvement or stabilization. To the best of our knowledge, we provide as well for the first time data in regard to the im levofolinate treatment dosage.

Introduction

Hereditary folate malabsorption (HFM; OMIM 229050) is a rare autosomal recessive disorder caused by impaired active folate transport across membranes and into the central nervous system due to loss-of-function mutations in proton-coupled folate transporter (PCFT) (Kronn and Goldman 2008; Qiu et al. 2006; Zhao et al. 2009). The severe systemic folate deficiency concomitant with impaired transport of folate across the blood-choroid plexus-brain barrier represents the pathophysiological basis of the disease and results in a marked deficiency of cerebrospinal fluid (CSF) folate (Zhao et al. 2007, 2009; Geller et al. 2002).

Infants with HFM come to medical attention in early infancy when they present with non-specific systemic findings such as failure to thrive, feeding difficulties, diarrhea, megaloblastic anemia, and/or pancytopenia in the context of really low baseline serum folate concentrations (Kronn and Goldman 2008; Zhao et al. 2017). One of the most unique aspects of the disease is an immune deficiency which occurs in a setting of significant hypogammaglobulinemia resulting in infections with unusual organisms (Zhao et al. 2017; Borzutzky et al. 2009). Neurologic symptoms may present concomitantly or develop progressively without adequate treatment (Kronn and Goldman 2008; Zhao et al. 2017). Developmental delay, peripheral neuropathy, movement disorder, behavioral issues, and seizures have been observed in the vast majority of reported

Communicated by: William Ross Wilcox, MD, PhD

E. Manea · P. Gissen · S. Batzios (✉)
Department of Paediatric Metabolic Medicine, Great Ormond Street Hospital, London, UK
e-mail: spyros.batzios@gmail.com

S. Pope · S.J. Heales
Neurometabolic Unit, National Hospital for Neurology and Neurosurgery, London, UK

S.J. Heales
Department of Chemical Pathology, Great Ormond Street Hospital, London, UK

patients with HFM (Kronn and Goldman 2008; Zhao et al. 2017). Diagnosis is suspected on the basis of the above-mentioned clinical features and hematological findings, which should prompt the clinician to measure CSF 5-methyltetrahydrofolate (5-MTHF) levels which are usually very low or undetectable. Confirmation of the diagnosis is made by detection of biallelic disease causing mutations in the SLC46A1 gene.

Early diagnosis is important for the initiation of treatment. Previous literature reports recommend high doses of oral or intramuscular (im) 5-formyltetrahydrofolate (5-formylTHF), also known as folinic acid, aiming to improve or normalize 5-MTHF CSF levels before irreversible damage occurs (Kronn and Goldman 2008; Zhao et al. 2017). Nevertheless, those levels are difficult to achieve even in patients who have been receiving high doses of parenteral folinic acid (Torres et al. 2015). The active isomer of 5-formylTHF, also known as levofolinic acid, is as well available for administration. Anecdotal observations suggest that the active isomer might be more effective, especially in patients with neurological involvement and refractory seizures (Kronn and Goldman 2008). Herein we report three cases of patients with HFM who received im levofolinate treatment. Follow-up assessment with repeated lumbar punctures has shown a normalization of their trough 5-MTHF levels and stabilization of clinical features and brain MRI findings. Trough CSF 5-MTHF levels were measured 24 h post-levofolinate dose and prior to the next dose. Based on achieving normal CSF 5-MTHF results, to the best of our knowledge, we provide for the first time data in regard to the im levofolinate treatment dosage.

Case Presentation 1

The first patient is the only son of non-consanguineous parents of British origin, born at term following an uneventful pregnancy. This patient's clinical features were previously reported (Shin et al. 2011). He presented to his local hospital at 2 months of age with failure to thrive, pallor, and diarrhea. He was diagnosed with Pneumocystis jiroveci pneumonia. Initial work-up showed megaloblastic anemia, neutropenia, undetectable serum folate with normal vitamin B12 levels. IgG levels were normal but IgA and IgM levels were low. Following initial intravenous folinic acid replacement patient was discharged home on oral folic acid supplementation of 1.5 mg/day and immunoglobulin replacement therapy.

Follow-up at 6 months of age demonstrated macrocytic anemia, neutropenia, low serum/red cell folate, and no specific immunodeficiency abnormalities. The dose of oral folic acid was increased. At the age of 13 months the patient showed developmental arrest, movement disorder,

and signs of central motor neuron involvement. The oral folic acid supplementation was again increased. At this point patient had a normal brain MRI and a lumbar puncture was unsuccessful. Even on high doses of oral folic acid patient continued to have the same clinical features and hematologic abnormalities. Based on the above constellation of findings HFM was suspected. Undetectable CSF 5-MTHF levels were in agreement with the clinical diagnosis (Table 1). Genetic analysis confirmed the diagnosis and patient was found to be compound heterozygous, with a mutant allele from his mother (c.204-205delCC) in exon 1 resulting in a frameshift starting at position N68 with early termination of translation, and a mutant allele from his father located in exon 2 (c.1004 C>A) resulting in an A335D loss-of-function point mutation (Shin et al. 2011). At this point patient was started on im folinic acid which led to an improvement of his clinical features; nevertheless, CSF 5-MTHF levels remained suboptimal.

Annual reviews showed delay of gross/fine motor skills, significant visual perceptual difficulty as well as slow witnessed continuous acquisition of skills with support. At the age of 5½ years the patient developed sudden mood swings and drop attacks. He also started having episodes of generalized tonic-clonic seizures, on a weekly basis, and complex partial seizures on a daily basis (up to 30 episodes/day). Epileptic activity was confirmed with an EEG. Patient was started on antiepileptic treatment and im levofolinic acid was introduced. Results from a repeat lumbar puncture 1 year following the initiation of levofolinate shown normal levels of 5-MTHF and brain MRI. Currently, at the age of 10 years the patient remains seizure free for 3½ years without any antiepileptic medication and continues to have a normal 5-MTHF CSF level. To date, no local or systemic complications have emerged from the use of im injections.

Case Presentation 2

Patient 2 is the first male child of non-consanguineous parents of Pakistani origin born at term after an uncomplicated pregnancy. He presented at 2 months of age with failure to thrive and irritability. On clinical examination patient presented subtle facial dysmorphism and hypospadias. Initial laboratory work-up showed severe pancytopenia requiring red blood cell and platelet transfusion. Plasma folate level was virtually zero and vitamin B12 was low. IM vitamin B12 and oral folic acid supplementation was started. Good progress was initially documented although plasma folate levels remained suboptimal and total plasma homocysteine was elevated. Vitamin B12 level normalized with im treatment within 2 months, however, patient was lost to follow-up.

Table 1 Biochemical and neuroimaging findings in Patient 1

Age	CSF 5-MTHF	Medication	Imaging
17 months	<10 nmol/L ref. 72–305	Folinic acid, 5 mg/day, im (0.4 mg/kg/day)	Normal intracranial appearances
2 years 6 months	19 nmol/L (trough level) ref. 52–178	Folinic acid, 12 mg/day, im (0.8 mg/kg/day)	Non-specific myelination delay and lack of white matter bulk
3 years	31 nmol/L (trough level) ref. 52–178	Folinic acid, 12 mg/day, im (0.71 mg/kg/day)	Subcortical white matter of bilateral cerebral hemispheres better myelinated, unchanged lack of white matter bulk, no other intracranial changes
5 years	14 nmol/L (trough level) ref. 52–178	Folinic acid, 12 mg/day, im (0.6 mg/kg/day)	No abnormality demonstrated
6 years	17 nmol/L (trough level) ref. 72–172	Sodium levofolinate, 15 mg/day, im (0.61 mg/kg/day)	Normal intracranial and intra-spinal appearances
7 years	52 nmol/L (trough level) ref. 72–172	Sodium levofolinate, 20 mg/day, im (0.78 mg/kg/day)	Normal intracranial and intra-spinal appearances
10 years	62 nmol/L (trough level) ref. 46–160	Sodium levofolinate, 50 mg/day, im (1.13 mg/kg/day)	

Six months later, while in Pakistan, patient underwent brain CT scan, following new onset epilepsy. The scan demonstrated basal ganglia calcification and cerebral atrophy. At the age of 17 months the patient was admitted to PICU because of status epilepticus. Clinical examination revealed truncal hypotonia, movement disorder, and dystonia with poor visual interaction. EEG at that point showed hypsarrhythmia. Because of the above constellation of findings a lumbar puncture for a full CSF work-up was done. The CSF 5-MTHF was undetectable with the rest of findings within normal range. Gene mutation analysis confirmed the diagnosis of hereditary folate malabsorption due to a homozygous c.198C>A, p.Cys66* mutation causing a premature stop codon. This mutation has been previously reported in literature in a patient who was compound heterozygous (Min et al. 2008), but not in a homozygous state. Patient was started initially on oral folinic acid supplementation and 4 months later on im daily injections which led to clinical and biochemical improvement (Table 2 and Fig. 1).

Although on im folinic acid therapy, patient's neurologic progress was turbulent with recurrent PICU admissions for status epilepticus, development of infantile spasms and subsequently myoclonic jerks which required combined antiepileptic drugs. At the age of 2 the patient was started im levofolinate treatment which led to the normalization of his 5-MTHF levels. Currently, at the age of 5 years the patient continues to have significant neurological deficit and intractable seizures, auditory and visual impairment, and medication controlled movement disorder.

Case Presentation 3

Patient 3 is the younger brother of Patient 2. Parents have declined antenatal testing. The pregnancy was uneventful and patient was delivered at term in good condition.

The investigations which were carried out on the second day of life showed mild thrombocytopenia, with normal serum folate, red cell folate, and homocysteine. CSF 5-MTHF level was nevertheless really low. Genetic analysis confirmed the presence of the same mutation as in the case of his brother in homozygous state. Levofolinate treatment was started at a dose of 5 mg/kg/day as one intramuscular daily dose (Table 3). Trough CSF 5-MTHF levels at 1 month of age showed normalization. Dose per kg decreased with age because of increasing weight and follow-up assessment at the age of 6 months showed low CSF 5-MTHF levels. Dose was increased to 4.5 mg/kg/day. The neurologic progress and the brain MRI findings are normal up to date.

Discussion

HFM is a rare autosomal recessive condition affecting folate metabolism. So far 37 families have been described worldwide, out of which 30 have as well genetic confirmation (Zhao et al. 2007, 2017; Diop-Bove et al. 2013; Mahadeo et al. 2011; Atabay et al. 2010). Our patients were found to have mutations already described in literature as pathogenic (Shin et al. 2011; Min et al. 2008). HFM is a

Table 2 Biochemical and neuroimaging findings in Patient 2

Age	CSF 5-MTHF	Medication	Imaging
17 months	<10 nmol/L ref. 72–305	Folinic acid, 10 mg/day, oral	
19 months	<10 nmol/L (peak sample) ref. 72–305	Folinic acid, 30 mg/day, oral	
21 months	11 nmol/L (peak sample) ref. 72–305	Folinic acid, 15 mg/day, im (2.5 mg/kg/day)	Ponto-cerebellar hypoplasia in addition to generalized lack of cerebral volume and myelination, bilateral symmetrical mature hemorrhagic infarction of the basal ganglia, symmetrical periventricular, and deep white matter change over the frontal lobes (Fig. 1)
2 years	31 nmol/L (trough level) ref. 52–178	Sodium levofolinate, 20 mg/day, im (1.3 mg/kg/day)	
2 years 10 months	50 nmol/L (trough level) ref. 52–178	Sodium levofolinate, 50 mg/day, im (3.3 mg/kg/day)	
4 years 6 months	106 nmol/L (trough level) ref. 52–178	Sodium levofolinate, 40 mg/day, im (1.6 mg/kg/day)	No progression of prominent white matter changes and ponto-cerebellar volume reduction

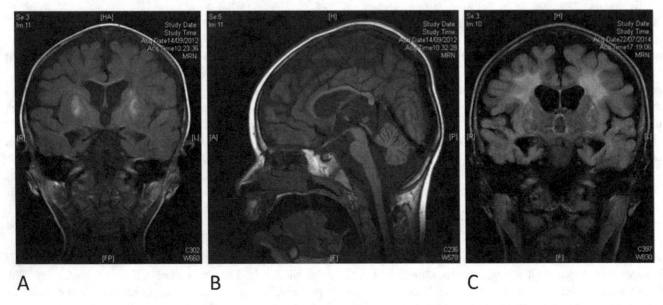

Fig. 1 MRI brain T1 weighted image showing basal ganglia calcifications (**a**), ponto-cerebellar hypoplasia, (**b**) T2 weighted image, (**c**) showing white matter changes over the frontal lobes

multisystemic disease, which emphasizes the major role of folate in different tissues and organs. Patients' clinical features have been recently summarized (Erlacher et al. 2015). Findings include poor feeding, faltering growth, megaloblastic anemia or even pancytopenia, diarrhea, immune dysfunction, and neurological manifestations with progressive deterioration (Kronn and Goldman 2008; Erlacher et al. 2015; Kishimoto et al. 2014). In our small cohort, Patient 1 and 2 had typical features of the disease, which in combination with low 5-MTHF led to the diagnosis of HFM. The abnormal findings on brain MRI

of patient 2 include calcification of the basal ganglia. Intracranial calcifications have been reported in other patients with HFM, typically presenting in the cortex or basal ganglia (Geller et al. 2002; Ahmad et al. 2015; Wang et al. 2015).

There have been no formal studies assessing the different folate formulations, dosing, and routes of administration that provide an evidence based regimen for optimal treatment. Most publications agree that parenteral administration of folinic acid is the only effective treatment for HFM. Even though anemia, immune dysfunction, and

Table 3 Biochemical and neuroimaging findings in Patient 3

Age	CSF 5-MTHF	Medication	Imaging
Day 2	12 nmol/L ref. 72–305	Sodium levofolinate, 15 mg/day, im (5 mg/kg/day)	
1 month	140 nmol/L (trough level) ref. 72–305	Sodium levofolinate, 15 mg/day, im	Brain MRI – normal
6 months	30 nmol/L (trough level) ref. 72–305	Sodium levofolinate, 15 mg/day, im (2 mg/kg/day)	

gastrointestinal symptoms are reversible with the oral or parenteral administration of folinic acid and normalization of blood folate levels is easily achieved, it has been proven that CSF levels remain suboptimal (Zhao et al. 2017; Borzutzky et al. 2009; Torres et al. 2015; Min et al. 2008; Erlacher et al. 2015; Kishimoto et al. 2014; Wang et al. 2015). Thus, the major challenge remains to achieve normal CSF 5-MTHF levels for treatment of neurological disease (Zhao et al. 2017).

This paper presents for the first time evidence of the effective correction of trough CSF 5-MTHF levels using im levofolinate in three patients with HFM. Two out of three patients were treated initially with oral and/or parenteral folinic acid, the racemic stable form of folate, which led to correction of the systemic manifestations. Nevertheless, CSF folate levels remained unsatisfactory, below the age dependent values, which prompted us to use levofolinate, the pharmacologically active isomer of 5-formylTHF. Daily im administration of the medication led to the normalization of trough 5-MTHF levels in the CSF and those levels remain stable and within normal range so far. Brain MRI findings had been stabilized. Clinical features of patients remained stable as well, while Patient 1 had a significant improvement in regard to his seizure activity. Initial dose in each patient was decided based on trough CSF 5-MTHF levels, and previous dose of folinic acid in combination with current knowledge that the biologic impact of the active isomer is twice that of the racemic compound at the same dose (Kronn and Goldman 2008). Hence, by using the active isomer, we were able to deliver double the amount of folate that would be delivered in the case the same dose of the racemic isoform was used. As a general remark we would say that the dose of im levofolinate which is required for the normalization of trough 5-MTHF CSF levels seems to be higher in neonates and infants and decreases with increasing age. This could demonstrate a higher demand of folate at the beginning of life and is in accordance as well with the fact that CSF folate levels are much higher in infancy and decrease with the advancing age (Zhao et al. 2017). Nevertheless, this theory has to be confirmed and appropriate dosing can only be decided when data from more patients with HFM on im levofolinate treatment are available. In addition it should be emphasized that individual CSF 5-MTHF levels may be influenced by multiple factors such as growth spurts, infections, and medication. These factors may explain to some degree the variation observed in our patients. Therefore the treatment regime should always be interpreted with regard to the overall clinical outcome and not just the CSF 5-MTHF levels. Finally, our results are based on assessment of trough CSF 5-MTHF levels. This represents a limitation of the study as 5-MTHF levels could have a great variation during the day which would not be depicted with just a single measurement.

Finally, this paper describes the youngest patient diagnosed with HFM and treated on the second day of life. This patient had only mild thrombocytopenia without any additional systemic or neurological findings.

Our patients did not experience any local or systemic complications as a consequence of the im injections. However, lifelong daily im administration is challenging and development of alternative and effective route of administration would be welcomed by the families.

Take Home Message

Intramuscular levofolinate administration represents an alternative treatment option in HFM which seems to result in normal CSF 5-MTHF levels and improvement of clinical features.

Details of the Contribution of Authors

EM has written part of the paper.

PG has supervised and provided corrections for the paper.

SP has done the laboratory analysis and provided comments for the paper.

SJH has done the laboratory analysis and provided comments for the paper.

SB has supervised and written part of the paper.

Corresponding Author

Spyros Batzios, Consultant in Paediatric Metabolic Medicine.

Compliance with Ethics Guidelines

Conflict of Interest

Emanuela Manea, Paul Gissen, Simon Pope, Simon J. Heales, and Spyros Batzios declare that they have no conflict of interest.

Informed Consent

No experimental procedures were done in the human subjects which are reported in this paper so no ethical approval was required. All tests were done as part of the normal review of the patients. Parents gave informed consent for the publication of the paper.

Animal Rights

No animal is involved in this study.

This article does not contain any studies with human or animal subjects performed by the any of the authors.

References

Ahmad I, Mukhtar G, Iqbal J, Ali SW (2015) Hereditary folate malabsorption with extensive intracranial calcification. Indian Pediatr 52(1):67–68

Atabay B, Turker M, Ozer EA, Mahadeo K, Diop-Bove N, Goldman ID (2010) Mutation of the proton-coupled folate transporter gene (PCFT-SLC46A1) in Turkish siblings with hereditary folate malabsorption. Pediatr Hematol Oncol 27(8):614–619

Borzutzky A, Crompton B, Bergmann AK et al (2009) Reversible severe combined immunodeficiency phenotype secondary to a mutation of the proton-coupled folate transporter. Clin Immunol 133(3):287–294

Diop-Bove N, Jain M, Scaglia F, Goldman ID (2013) A novel deletion mutation in the proton-coupled folate transporter (PCFT; SLC46A1) in a Nicaraguan child with hereditary folate malabsorption. Gene 527(2):673–674

Erlacher M, Grünert SC, Cseh A et al (2015) Reversible pancytopenia and immunodeficiency in a patient with hereditary folate malabsorption. Pediatr Blood Cancer 62(6):1091–1094

Geller J, Kronn D, Jayabose S, Sandoval C (2002) Hereditary folate malabsorption: family report and review of the literature. Medicine (Baltimore) 81(1):51–68

Kishimoto K, Kobayashi R, Sano H et al (2014) Impact of folate therapy on combined immunodeficiency secondary to hereditary folate malabsorption. Clin Immunol 153(1):17–22

Kronn D, Goldman ID (2008) Hereditary folate malabsorption. In: Pagon RA, Adam MP, Ardinger HH, Wallace SE, Amemiya A, Bean LJH, Bird TD, Ledbetter N, Mefford HC, Smith RJH, Stephens K (eds) GeneReviews®. University of Washington, Seattle, pp 1993–2017. http://www.ncbi.nlm.nih.gov/books/NBK1673/. Updated 2017 [Internet]

Mahadeo KM, Diop-Bove N, Ramirez SI et al (2011) Prevalence of a loss-of-function mutation in the proton-coupled folate transporter gene (PCFT-SLC46A1) causing hereditary folate malabsorption in Puerto Rico. J Pediatr 159(4):623–627

Min SH, Oh SY, Karp GI, Poncz M, Zhao R, Goldman ID (2008) The clinical course and genetic defect in the PCFT gene in a 27-year-old woman with hereditary folate malabsorption. J Pediatr 153 (3):435–437

Qiu A, Jansen M, Sakaris A et al (2006) Identification of an intestinal folate transporter and the molecular basis for hereditary folate malabsorption. Cell 127(5):917–928

Shin DS, Mahadeo K, Min SH et al (2011) Identification of novel mutations in the proton-coupled folate transporter (PCFT-SLC46A1) associated with hereditary folate malabsorption. Mol Genet Metab 103(1):33–37

Torres A, Newton SA, Crompton B et al (2015) CSF 5-methyltetrahydrofolate serial monitoring to guide treatment of congenital folate malabsorption due to proton-coupled folate transporter (PCFT) deficiency. JIMD Rep 24:91–96

Wang Q, Li X, Ding Y, Liu Y, Qin Y, Yang Y (2015) The first Chinese case report of hereditary folate malabsorption with a novel mutation on SLC46A1. Brain and Development 37(1):163–167

Zhao R, Min SH, Qiu A et al (2007) The spectrum of mutations in the PCFT gene, coding for an intestinal folate transporter, that are the basis for hereditary folate malabsorption. Blood 110(4):1147–1152

Zhao R, Min SH, Wang Y, Campanella E, Low PS, Goldman ID (2009) A role for the proton-coupled folate transporter (PCFT-SLC46A1) in folate receptor-mediated endocytosis. J Biol Chem 284(7):4267–4274

Zhao R, Aluri S, Goldman ID (2017) The proton-coupled folate transporter (PCFT-SLC46A1) and the syndrome of systemic and cerebral folate deficiency of infancy: hereditary folate malabsorption. Mol Asp Med 53:57–72

JIMD Reports
DOI 10.1007/8904_2017_41

RESEARCH REPORT

The Prevalence of PMM2-CDG in Estonia Based on Population Carrier Frequencies and Diagnosed Patients

Mari-Anne Vals · Sander Pajusalu · Mart Kals · Reedik Mägi · Katrin Õunap

Received: 06 May 2017 / Revised: 10 June 2017 / Accepted: 16 June 2017 / Published online: 07 July 2017
© SSIEM and Springer-Verlag Berlin Heidelberg 2017

Abstract PMM2-CDG (MIM#212065) is the most common type of congenital disorders of glycosylation (CDG) caused by mutations in *PMM2* (MIM#601785). In Estonia, five patients from three families have been diagnosed with PMM2-CDG. Our aim was to evaluate the presence of different PMM2-CDG-causing mutations in a population-based cohort and to calculate the expected frequency of PMM2-CDG in Estonia. Also, we analyzed the prevalence of PMM2-CDG based on our patient group data. To calculate the expected frequency of PMM2-CDG, we used the whole genome sequencing data of 2,244 participants from biobank of the Estonian Genome Center, University of Tartu. Nineteen individuals carried mutated *PMM2* alleles and altogether, five different mutations were identified. The observed carrier frequency for all *PMM2* disease-causing mutations was thus 1/118, and for the most frequent mutation p.R141H, 1/224. The expected frequency of the disease in Estonian population is 1/77,000. It is comparable to the current prevalence of PMM2-CDG for the less than 18 years age group, which is 1/79,000. In conclusion, the frequency of PMM2-CDG in Estonia is lower than in other European populations reported thus far. We demonstrate that biobank data can be useful for gaining new information about the epidemiology of the PMM2-CDG.

Introduction

PMM2-CDG (MIM#212065) is the most common type of congenital disorders of glycosylation (CDG), and is inherited in an autosomal recessive pattern. There are at least 1,000 diagnosed PMM2-CDG patients worldwide, but the number is likely increasing as the awareness of CDG is growing.

PMM2 (MIM#601785) is located in chromosomal region 16p13 (Martinsson et al. 1994), with at least 117 disease-causing mutations listed in the Human Gene Mutation Database (HGMD® Professional) from BIOBASE Corporation (Stenson et al. 2009), and 97 of them are missense mutations. In most cases, PMM-CDG patients are compound heterozygotes, and there are no reports describing the homozygosity of the most frequent mutation p.R141H because it is probably embryonically lethal (Matthijs et al. 1998). The homozygous state of other mutations like p.F119L, p.Y64C, p.D65Y, p.P113L, p.N216I, p.Y106F, p.F183S, and p.T237M has been described by different authors (Matthijs et al. 2000; Neumann et al. 2003; Najmabadi et al. 2011; Perez et al. 2011).

The population-based biobank of the Estonian Genome Center at the University of Tartu (EGCUT) contains almost 52,000 samples of the adult population (aged ≥18 years), which closely reflects the age, sex, and geographical distribution of the Estonian population, making it a valuable resource for population-based genetic studies (Leitsalu et al. 2015). Regarding clinical care, there is only

Communicated by: Eva Morava, MD PhD

M.-A. Vals (✉) · S. Pajusalu · K. Õunap
Department of Clinical Genetics, United Laboratories, Tartu University Hospital, Tartu, Estonia
e-mail: mari-anne.vals@kliinikum.ee

M.-A. Vals · S. Pajusalu · K. Õunap
Department of Clinical Genetics, Institute of Clinical Medicine, University of Tartu, Tartu, Estonia

M.-A. Vals
Children's Clinic, Tartu University Hospital, Tartu, Estonia

M. Kals · R. Mägi
Estonian Genome Center, University of Tartu, Tartu, Estonia

one center in Estonia at the Tartu University Hospital (TUH) that consults the patients suffering from inborn errors of metabolism. Since 2012, CDG screening (serum transferrin isoelectric focusing, TIEF) is performed at TUH on requests made by clinicians from the whole country. Thus, it is highly likely that all patients diagnosed with CDG in Estonia have been clinically followed up in TUH.

Several reports describe different *PMM2* mutations and their frequencies in larger cohorts of PMM2-CDG patients, but to our knowledge, only one report has estimated the disease frequency based on allele frequencies among healthy individuals (Schollen et al. 2000). Our aim was to evaluate the presence of different PMM2-CDG-causing mutations in a population-based cohort and to calculate the expected frequency of PMM2-CDG in Estonia. Also, we analyzed the prevalence of PMM2-CDG based on our patient group data.

Methods

Population Cohort

Whole genome sequencing (WGS) data of 2,244 geographically distributed individuals (selected randomly by county of birth) from EGCUT were available. WGS samples were sequenced at the Broad Institute (Cambridge, MA, USA) following a PCR-free sample preparation. Libraries were sequenced on the Illumina HiSeq X Ten (Illumina, San Diego, CA, USA) with the use of 150 bp paired-end reads to 30× mean coverage with a median insert size of 400 bp ± 25%.

All variants identified in the *PMM2* were extracted and alleles listed as disease-causing according to HGMD were counted to estimate pathogenic allele frequencies. In addition, all other protein-altering variants were evaluated for possible additional novel disease-causing mutations.

Patient Cohort

Five patients from three families (Table 1) have been diagnosed with PMM2-CDG in Estonia. All of them have European ancestry and their parents are unrelated Estonians,

except for one parent who is French. All patients showed positive TIEF type 1 profile on screening and PMM2-CDG was molecularly confirmed with different DNA sequencing approaches.

Statistical Methods

According to census in 2011, there are 1.29 million enumerated residents in Estonia and 18.4% of them are children, defined as age less than 18 years. To calculate the expected disease frequency, we used the assumption of p. R141H homozygotes being embryonically lethal (Matthijs et al. 1998). Thus, if q is the allele frequency of p.R141H and r the combined allele frequency for other identified mutations in our cohort, then $r^2 + 2qr$ denotes the expected disease frequency in the given population. For 95% confidence intervals (CI), test of given proportions (prop. test) was conducted in R version 3.2.3 (R Core Team 2016).

Results

Population Cohort

Out of 2,244 samples, 19 carried one mutated *PMM2* allele and altogether, five different mutations were identified: p. R141H (10 alleles), p.V231M (5 alleles), p.R239W (2 alleles), p.V67M and p.T237R (both 1 allele) (Table 2). In addition to disease-causing variants appearing in HGMD, no possibly pathogenic novel mutations were identified. Based on these results, the observed carrier frequency for all *PMM2* disease-causing mutations was 1/118 (95% CI 1/74–1/190) and for the most frequent mutation p.R141H, 1/224 (95% CI 1/118–1/441). Allele frequency of p.R141H (q) was 1/449 and of other mutations (r), 1/499. Based on these data, the expected frequency of the disease ($r^2 + 2qr$) in Estonian population is 1/77,000.

Patients

The five patients were born from 1998 to 2015. One patient died in the first week of life and one has reached adulthood. Thus, the current prevalence of PMM2-CDG can be calculated for the whole population (four cases) as 1/322,000 (95% CI 1/117,000–1/1,007,000) and for the less than 18 years age group (three cases), 1/79,000 (95% CI 1/25,000–1/306,000).

Discussion

Many reports from different European countries describe cohorts of patients diagnosed with PMM2-CDG. The

Table 1 PMM2-CDG genotypes in Estonia

PMM2-CDG genotypes	Number of patients	Phenotype
p.R141H/p.V231M	1	Severe
p.R239W/p.V231M	3[a]	Mild
p.R123Q/p.V231M	1	Severe

[a] Siblings, described by Vals et al. (2017)

Table 2 Number of *PMM2* mutations identified in population cohort (2,244 individuals) and the diagnosed five patients (three families)

Mutation	Population cohort	Patients
p.V67M	1	–
p.R141H	10	1
p.V231M	5	3
p.T237R	1	–
p.R239W	2	1
p.R123Q	–	1

results give an overview about the frequencies of different mutations and genotypes, as well as their geographical distribution. p.R141H is the most commonly found mutation among molecularly confirmed Caucasian PMM2-CDG patients with prevalence ranging from 20.6 to 44% (Kjaergaard et al. 1998; Matthijs et al. 2000; Perez et al. 2011). Still, the population data have been only reported by Schollen et al. who studied p.R141H and p.F119L frequencies among Dutch neonates and Danish blood donors (Schollen et al. 2000). They showed that the carrier frequency for p.R141H is 1/72 and the expected disease frequency is 1/20,000 in these populations.

The Estonian Biobank represents 5% of Estonian adults and offers a unique database for research and population-based studies (Leitsalu et al. 2015). The data of 2,244 individuals revealed five different mutations with a combined carrier frequency of 1/118 for all mutations. The carrier frequency for p.R141H was 1/224. Compared to our results, the Dutch and Danish pooled data show a three times higher p.R141H frequency. Carrier frequency for other mutations is estimated to be 1/300 to 1/400 (Schollen et al. 2000) which in our population ranges from 1/448 to 1/2,244 depending on the mutation.

To our knowledge, there are no reports about the patients homozygous for the mutations identified in our cohort. Only the homozygosity of p.R141H has been shown to be absent, as it is probably lethal (Matthijs et al. 1998). By excluding p.R141H homozygotes, the expected frequency of PMM2-CDG in the Estonian population according to the modified Hardy–Weinberg equilibrium is 1/77,000. The frequency might be somewhat lower, as we have not considered the possibility that some of the recombinants of detected mutations are incompatible with life. If we compare the frequency with our population size and its age-specific distribution, there should be up to 16 people, including 3 children, with PMM2-CDG in Estonia.

So far, we have molecularly confirmed the PMM2-CDG in five children from three families. They are compound heterozygotes with four different previously described missense mutations. Undeniably, because of the small number of patients, it is difficult to draw any conclusions

about the characteristic genotypes among our patients as well as to compare them with other countries, but they all have p.V231M in one allele and only one patient has p.R141H in the other allele. Based on their genotypes, our hypothesis was that the most frequent *PMM2* mutation among Estonians is p.V231M. However, similarly to the other reports, the most frequently found mutation among biobank participants was p.R141H (56%) and p.V231M was the second most common mutation (23%). p.R239W was also represented in the population cohort, but p.R123Q was not. It might be explained by the fact that the allele with p.R123Q is inherited from the parent with French origin and the mutation is not geographically characteristic of Estonia. In our population cohort, we also did not find p.F119L, which is the second most common mutation among the South-Scandinavian population (Kjaergaard et al. 1998; Bjursell et al. 2000).

The prevalence of PMM2-CDG in Estonia in the whole population calculated by patient data was much lower, 1/322,000. We believe that the prevalence must be higher as the disease has not been diagnosed in any adult patients. Therefore, based on the data about the expected frequency of the disease, there should be undiagnosed patients with PMM2-CDG in Estonia whether due to patients not surviving into adulthood or due to the possible presence of undiagnosed individuals with mild phenotype. Although the availability of diagnostic tests is good in Estonia, congenital metabolic diseases, including CDG, are less likely to be considered and investigated by clinicians among the adult patients and CDG screening with serum TIEF serves mainly children. This is supported by the fact that three out of the five patients in Estonia were diagnosed with PMM2-CDG during infancy and that two other patients with a mild clinical presentation got their diagnosis as adolescents after the diagnosis of their youngest sibling (Vals et al. 2017). A similar age distribution favoring the diagnosis in children was showed by Matthijs et al. (2000). Therefore we also calculated the prevalence among children. As one patient has reached adulthood, the prevalence in the less than 18 years age group is 1/79,000, which is similar to the expected frequency of PMM2-CDG in Estonia based on population allele frequencies.

In conclusion, we showed that the frequency of PMM2-CDG in Estonia is lower than in other European populations reported thus far. We have also demonstrated that population cohort data give useful new information about the epidemiology of the PMM2-CDG.

Acknowledgements This work was supported and funded by the Estonian Research Council grant PUT355, EU H2020 grant 692145, Estonian Research Council Grant IUT20-60, IUT24-6 and European Union through the European Regional Development Fund Project No. 2014-2020.4.01.15-0012 GENTRANSMED.

Author Disclosure Statement

The authors declare no potential conflicts of interest with respect to the authorship and/or publication of this article.

Concise One-Sentence Take-Home Message

The expected frequency of the PMM2-CDG in Estonian population is 1/77,000.

General Rules

Details of the Contributions of Individual Authors

Mari-Anne Vals – performed serum transferrin isoelectric focusing to four patients, analyzed the population cohort data, performed statistical analysis, and compiled the manuscript.

Sander Pajusalu – analyzed the population cohort data, performed statistical analysis, coordinated analysis between different centers, and compiled the manuscript.

Mart Kals – analyzed biobank data, including quality control and compiled the manuscript.

Reedik Mägi – analyzed biobank data and compiled the manuscript.

Katrin Õunap – planned the study, diagnosed PMM2-CDG patients, coordinated work between different centers, and compiled the manuscript.

Correspondent and Guarantor

Mari-Anne Vals.

A Competing Interest Statement

The authors Mari-Anne Vals, Sander Pajusalu, Mart Kals, Reedik Mägi, and Katrin Õunap declare no potential conflicts of interest with respect to the authorship and/or publication of this article.

Details of Funding

This work was supported and funded by the Estonian Research Council grant PUT355, EU H2020 grant 692145, Estonian Research Council Grant IUT20-60, IUT24-6 and European Union through the European Regional Development Fund Project No. 2014-2020.4.01.15-0012 GEN-TRANSMED.

Details of Ethics Approval

This study was approved by the Research Ethics Committee of the University of Tartu (181/T-16, 20.04.2009 and 235/M-13, 17.03.2014). All participants in Estonian Biobank have signed a broad consent for using their data for research, and we also have an approval from the local ethics committee to use the omics data of gene donors of Estonian Biobank for genetic research (approval 234/T-12 for "Omics for health: an integrated approach to understand and predict human disease").

A Patient Consent Statement

Informed consent was obtained from the parents of the five patients.

References

Bjursell C, Erlandson A, Nordling M et al (2000) PMM2 mutation spectrum, including 10 novel mutations, in a large CDG type 1A family material with a focus on Scandinavian families. Hum Mutat 16:395–400

Kjaergaard S, Skovby F, Schwartz M (1998) Absence of homozygosity for predominant mutations in PMM2 in Danish patients with carbohydrate-deficient glycoprotein syndrome type 1. Eur J Hum Genet 6:331–336

Leitsalu L, Haller T, Esko T et al (2015) Cohort profile: Estonian biobank of the Estonian Genome Center, University of Tartu. Int J Epidemiol 44:1137–1147

Martinsson T, Bjursell C, Stibler H et al (1994) Linkage of a locus for carbohydrate-deficient glycoprotein syndrome type I (CDG1) to chromosome 16p, and linkage disequilibrium to microsatellite marker D16S406. Hum Mol Genet 3:2037–2042

Matthijs G, Schollen E, Van Schaftingen E, Cassiman JJ, Jaeken J (1998) Lack of homozygotes for the most frequent disease allele in carbohydrate-deficient glycoprotein syndrome type 1A. Am J Hum Genet 62:542–550

Matthijs G, Schollen E, Bjursell C et al (2000) Mutations in PMM2 that cause congenital disorders of glycosylation, type Ia (CDG-Ia). Hum Mutat 16:386–394

Najmabadi H, Hu H, Garshasbi M et al (2011) Deep sequencing reveals 50 novel genes for recessive cognitive disorders. Nature 478:57–63

Neumann LM, von Moers A, Kunze J, Blankenstein O, Marquardt T (2003) Congenital disorder of glycosylation type 1a in a macrosomic 16-month-old boy with an atypical phenotype and homozygosity of the N216I mutation. Eur J Pediatr 162:710–713

Perez B, Briones P, Quelhas D et al (2011) The molecular landscape of phosphomannose mutase deficiency in iberian peninsula: identification of 15 population-specific mutations. JIMD Rep 1:117–123

R Core Team (2016) R: a language and environment for statistical computing. In: Book R: a language and environment for statistical computing. R Foundation for Statistical Computing, Vienna

Schollen E, Kjaergaard S, Legius E, Schwartz M, Matthijs G (2000) Lack of Hardy-Weinberg equilibrium for the most prevalent PMM2 mutation in CDG-Ia (congenital disorders of glycosylation type Ia). Eur J Hum Genet 8:367–371

Stenson PD, Mort M, Ball EV et al (2009) The human gene mutation database: 2008 update. Genome Med 1:13

Vals MA, Morava E, Teeaar K et al (2017) Three families with mild PMM2-CDG and normal cognitive development. Am J Med Genet A 173:1620–1624

JIMD Reports
DOI 10.1007/8904_2017_36

RESEARCH REPORT

Triheptanoin: A Rescue Therapy for Cardiogenic Shock in Carnitine-acylcarnitine Translocase Deficiency

Sidharth Mahapatra · Amitha Ananth · Nancy Baugh ·
Mihaela Damian · Gregory M. Enns

Received: 16 March 2017 / Revised: 31 May 2017 / Accepted: 07 June 2017 / Published online: 09 July 2017
© SSIEM and Springer-Verlag Berlin Heidelberg 2017

Abstract Carnitine-acylcarnitine translocase (CACT) deficiency is a rare long-chain fatty acid oxidation disorder (LC-FAOD) with high mortality due to cardiomyopathy or lethal arrhythmia. Triheptanoin (UX007), an investigational drug composed of synthetic medium odd-chain triglycerides, is a novel therapy in development for LC-FAOD patients. However, cases of its safe and efficacious use to reverse severe heart failure in CACT deficiency are limited. Here, we present a detailed report of an infant with CACT deficiency admitted in metabolic crisis that progressed into severe cardiogenic shock who was successfully treated by triheptanoin. The child was managed, thereafter, on triheptanoin until her death at 3 years of age from a cardiopulmonary arrest in the setting of acute respiratory illness superimposed on chronic hypercarbic respiratory failure.

Communicated by: Manuel Schiff

S. Mahapatra (✉)
Division of Critical Care, Department of Pediatrics, University of
Nebraska Medical Center, Omaha, NE 68198, USA
e-mail: smahapatra@childrensomaha.org

A. Ananth
Pediatric Neurology, Brain and Spine Institute, Providence Health and
Services, Portland, OR 97225, USA

N. Baugh
Department of Clinical Nutrition, Lucile Packard Children's Hospital,
Stanford, Palo Alto, CA 94304, USA

M. Damian
Division of Critical Care, Department of Pediatrics, Stanford
University Medical Center, Palo Alto, CA 94304, USA

G.M. Enns
Division of Medical Genetics, Department of Pediatrics, Stanford
University Medical Center, Palo Alto, CA 94304, USA

Introduction

Long-chain fatty acid oxidation disorders (LC-FAOD) are a group of autosomal recessive inborn errors of metabolism wherein genetic defects in specific mitochondrial enzymes lead to an inability to convert long-chain fatty acids to energy during periods of physiologic stress (Vockley et al. 2017). Amongst the most uncommon fatty acid oxidation disorders, carnitine-acylcarnitine translocase (CACT) deficiency is caused by mutations in *SLC25A20* (Rubio-Gozalbo et al. 2004). CACT is an essential component of the carnitine cycle and is responsible for the importation of long-chain fatty acids from the cytosol into mitochondria for energy production via beta oxidation (Pande and Murthy 1994; Vitoria et al. 2015). Clinical abnormalities occur secondary to energy deprivation and accumulation of potentially toxic long-chain fatty acid intermediates (Rubio-Gozalbo et al. 2004). CACT dysfunction causes hypoketotic hypoglycemia, hyperammonemia, and impairment of fatty acid-dependent tissues, including the heart, liver, and skeletal muscle. Presentation is typically early in life with a relatively severe course, although minor phenotypes have been reported (Pande and Murthy 1994).

Since the first report of CACT deficiency by Stanley and colleagues in 1992, approximately 55 cases have been reported in the medical literature (Stanley et al. 1992; Vitoria et al. 2015). Treatment has focused on dietary modification with frequent, carbohydrate-rich meals, avoidance of fasting, restriction of fat intake, and supplementation with medium chain triglycerides (MCT) (Spiekerkoetter et al. 2009). However, the mortality rate for CACT deficiency remains high (65%), with most deaths occurring in the first year of life due to cardiac complications (Bonnet et al. 1999; Vitoria et al. 2015). The most common cardiac manifestation is cardiomyopathy, but

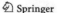

fatalities are more often reported due to conduction defects and arrhythmias (Bonnet et al. 1999). For patients with CACT deficiency and concomitant cardiac disease, current treatment options are limited to supportive care.

Triheptanoin (UX007) is an investigational drug composed of synthetic medium chain fatty acid which has been used on a compassionate or emergency basis in patients with LC-FAOD and severe cardiomyopathy (Roe and Brunengraber 2015; Vockley et al. 2015, 2016). Here, we present a detailed case of a patient with CACT deficiency and cardiomyopathy devolving into severe cardiogenic shock during a metabolic crisis. With failure of conventional treatments, including MCT and carnitine supplementation, we hypothesized that triheptanoin may arrest further cardiac deterioration and potentially lead to some recovery.

Case Report

The patient is a full-term female born to a 24-year-old G_1P_0 mother with no prenatal or antenatal complications via normal spontaneous vaginal delivery who initially presented with hypoketotic hypoglycemia (glucose 12 mg/dL, ref > 40 mg/dL) and hypothermia (95°F, ref: 97.5–99.3°F) at 23 h of life. Her ammonia and lactate peaked at 319 μmol/L (ref: 64–107 μmol/L) and 4.1 mmol/L (ref < 2 mmol/L), respectively, at 52 h of life. The acylcarnitine profile demonstrated abnormal elevation of numerous long-chain acylcarnitine species, particularly palmitoyl- (16) and oleyl- (C18:1) acylcarnitine, suggestive of carnitine palmitoyltransferase II or CACT deficiency. SLC25A20 molecular analysis identified compound heterozygosity for a previously reported c.84delT mutation and a 506-kb deletion on chromosome 3p21.31 which includes the SLC25A20 gene (Eto et al. 2013, Haldeman-Englert et al. 2009, Hsu et al. 2001). On day of life (DOL) 5, she was started on MCT oil to supplement total parenteral nutrition (TPN) and maternal breast milk (MBM). She was discharged on a high MCT formula, maternal breast milk, a carbohydrate module, and additional MCT oil, providing 145 kcal/kg, 1.5 g/kg protein, 33.5% fat calories, 9.5% from long chain fats (LCFA), and 24% from MCT. Of note, her initial echocardiogram (ECHO) at 4 days of age already showed signs of biventricular hypertrophy but with normal systolic function, i.e. left ventricular ejection fraction (EF) 64% and shortening fraction (SF) 41% (ref_{EF}: 49–86%, ref_{SF}: 25–45%). Thus, she was actively followed by the cardiac failure team.

At 5 months, she presented with severe metabolic crisis with hyperammonemia (314 μmol/L) and acute kidney injury (AKI) (creatinine 1.0 mg/dL, ref: 0.2–0.4 mg/dL). By hospital day 3, despite nutritional support with high dextrose-containing TPN, her left ventricular EF and SF had decreased from normal to 33% and 20%, respectively. Her cardiac enzymes rose

dramatically with a creatine kinase-MB isoenzyme (CK-MB) of 119 ng/mL (ref < 1.7 ng/mL), troponin of 24 ng/mL (ref < 0.1 ng/mL), and pro-basic natriuretic peptide (pro-BNP) >30,000 pg/mL (ref < 300 pg/mL). Associated arrhythmias (ectopy, diffuse ST changes, left bundle branch block, and QT_c prolongation >550 ms) ensued resulting in cardiogenic shock, necessitating veno-arterial extra-corporal membrane oxygenation (VA-ECMO) for 8 days. Upon recovery from this episode, her cardiac function returned to baseline, i.e. EF 73% and SF 45%. She was discharged on a high MCT formula, infant formula, a carbohydrate module, and additional MCT oil, providing 121 kcal/kg, 1.4 g/kg protein, 37% fat calories, 8.4% from LCFA, and 28.6% from MCT.

At 10 months of age, she suffered another severe metabolic crisis secondary to urinary tract infection and gastroenteritis requiring admission to the pediatric intensive care unit (PICU) for metabolic management and aggressive fluid resuscitation due to moderate dehydration secondary to emesis and diarrhea (stool output up to 30 mL/kg/day in the first 3 days of hospitalization). To provide sufficient calories, total parenteral nutrition (TPN) was started (15% dextrose, 1.2 g/kg amino acids) with continuation of enteral MCT oil, providing 107 kcal/kg/day, MCT providing 21% of total calories. She slowly improved clinically and enteral feedings were initiated on day 5 of hospitalization with gradual advancement to bolus feeds and discontinuation of TPN. She was thereafter transferred to the acute care ward.

However, on hospital day 8, she was transferred back to the PICU for dehydration from continued diarrhea (stool output >10 mL/kg/day) and oliguric renal failure (creatinine 0.9 mg/dL). Despite appropriate fluid and caloric management (restarted TPN with 10% dextrose, 0.7 g/kg protein, enteral MCT oil, providing 82 kcal/kg/day, with MCT providing 32% of total calories), she developed severe cardiogenic shock within 48 h with extreme tachycardia (>200/min) and hypotension. She had deep ST-depression with elevated cardiac enzymes, i.e. CK-MB and troponin at 97.7 ng/mL and 17.2 ng/mL, respectively. Her pro-BNP was >30,000 pg/mL, lactate peaked at 6.2 mmol/L, and creatinine peaked at 1.2 (Table 1). With myocardial ischemia, a strategy of using multiple low-dose dose vasoactive agents was adopted, including calcium chloride up to 7 mg/kg/h, dopamine up to 7 μg/kg/min, epinephrine up to 0.05 μg/kg/min, and dobutamine up to 7 μg/kg/min, targeting a mean arterial pressure of 50 mmHg, in conjunction with a beta-blocker (esmolol up to 150 μg/kg/min) targeting a heart rate <150/min to optimize cardiac output. She was also started on stress-dose steroids at 50 mg/m²/day.

Her overall dismal prognosis made her a poor ECMO candidate. On hospital day 13 (EF 24.9%, SF 12.4%, CK-MB 107 ng/mL, troponin 39.9 ng/mL) after obtaining authorization from the Food & Drug Administration (FDA), the Institutional Review Board (IRB), and parental consent,

Table 1 Laboratory test results before and after triheptanoin therapy

	Reference range	Admission to hospital	Transfer to PICU	Cardiogenic shock	Initiation of triheptanoin	After 72 h triheptanoin
Day of hospitalization	–	1	8	10	13	16
Ammonia	<30 μmol/L	143	241	52	40	32
Lactate	<2 mmol/L	0.6	2.8	3.2	1.8	1.9
Creatinine	0.1–0.6 mg/dL	0.4	0.9	1.2	0.9	0.5
Creatinine kinase, total	<250 U/L	N.C.[a]	N.C.	1,990	713	443
Creatinine kinase, MB	<1.7 ng/mL	N.C.	N.C.	97.7	107	24.7
Troponin	<0.1 ng/mL	N.C.	N.C.	17.2	40	7.9

[a] N.C. not checked

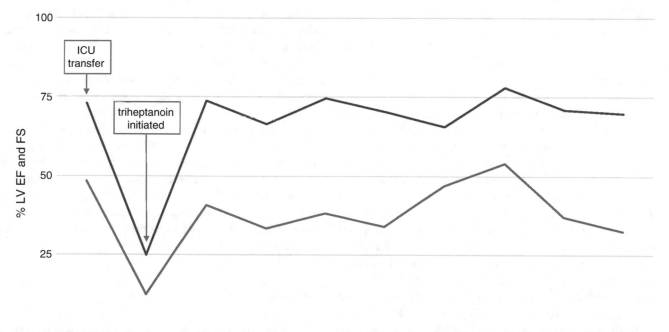

Day of Life	336	340	343	355	406	503	718	764	933	1139
——EF	72.9	24.9	73.7	66.6	74.8	70.4	65.6	78	71	70
——SF	48.2	12.4	40.6	33.3	38	34	47	54	37	32.6

Fig. 1 Cardiac function plotted over time. Prior to and even at admission to ICU, the patient maintained normal biventricular systolic and diastolic function, despite left ventricular hypertrophy. When she suffered cardiogenic shock, ejection fraction (EF) and shortening fraction (SF) both declined precipitously to approximately 25% and 12%, respectively. After 72 h of triheptanoin therapy, her EF and SF returned to baseline. She continued triheptanoin therapy till her death. Prior to death, her cardiac function was close to her baseline

MCT oil was stopped and triheptanoin was initiated via naso-jejunal tube at a dosage of 30 kcal/kg/day (34% of total calories). Three days after initiation of triheptanoin, a repeat ECHO showed normalization of left ventricular EF and SF (Fig. 1) and a >4-fold reduction in cardiac enzymes (Table 1). In the same time frame, all vasoactives were successfully weaned off.

Her enteral diet was advanced to include a very low fat elemental product, infant formula, and a protein module, which, with triheptanoin, provided 90 kcal/kg/day and 1.4 g/kg/day protein with 43% calories from fat, 11% from LCFA, and 32% from triheptanoin. Walnut oil was added as a source of essential fats. She was eventually extubated 18 days after triheptanoin initiation and discharged home a week later. ECHO prior to discharge showed biventricular hypertrophy with good biventricular systolic and diastolic function.

She continued triheptanoin after discharge; dosing was changed to four times a day for ease of administration. Since initiation of triheptanoin, she had two subsequent admissions, one for hyperammonemia due to acute gastroenteritis and a second for dehydration in the setting of *C. difficile* colitis. During both illnesses, her cardiac function remained stable. At her 20-month clinic visit, she was in overall good health and had developed the ability to sit independently. At 32 months of age, she was diagnosed with obstructive sleep apnea, hypoventilation, hypotonia and hypercarbic respiratory failure requiring noninvasive positive pressure ventilation.

At 3 years of age, she suffered a cardiac arrest precipitated by mucus plugging in the setting of a viral upper respiratory tract infection; care was withdrawn after admission due to devastating neurologic injury. ECHO performed after admission demonstrated no deterioration in function (Fig. 1, day of life 1,139: EF 70%, SF 32.6%). Additionally, her EKGs and rhythm strips showed normal sinus rhythm (NSR).

Discussion

Fatty acid oxidation generates energy during fasting and stress by directly supplying reducing equivalents for mitochondrial oxidative phosphorylation and providing acetyl-CoA to the tricarboxylic acid (TCA) cycle. Loss of this energy source along with impaired ketone body production during metabolic crisis leads to increased demand on the TCA cycle. Medium chain triglycerides are metabolized to the 2-carbon substrate acetyl-CoA that can enter the TCA cycle. In addition to two molecules of acetyl-CoA, triheptanoin provides a 3-carbon propionyl-CoA which can directly enter the TCA cycle as succinyl-CoA through the actions of propionyl-CoA carboxylase and methylmalonyl-CoA mutase (Roe and Mochel 2006). In this manner, triheptanoin provides appropriate substrate balance for the TCA cycle.

Triheptanoin, as treatment for fatty acid oxidation disorders, was first reported in the treatment of three patients with the cardiomyopathic form of very-long-chain acyl-CoA dehydrogenase deficiency (Roe et al. 2002). In these patients, congestive heart failure, rhabdomyolysis, and muscle weakness improved, as did the severity and frequency of metabolic decompensation. Results of a larger series of 20 patients with various long-chain fatty acid oxidation disorders treated with triheptanoin as part of a compassionate use protocol showed significant decreases in mean hospital days per year and hypoglycemia event rates. Of the 12 patients in the series that had cardiomyopathy at the start of triheptanoin therapy, 8 improved, 3 remained stable, and 1 required cardiac transplantation. The single CACT deficiency patient in this cohort had cardiomyopathy that improved, with ejection fraction increasing to 67% from 35% pre-treatment (Vockley et al.

2015). A subsequent case series of ten patients with LC-FAOD and acute heart failure in whom triheptanoin had been initiated for compassionate or emergency use demonstrated return of normal EF within 3 weeks of initiation; only two of these patients had CACT deficiency (Vockley et al. 2016). Now, a single-arm, open-label, multicenter Phase 2 trial has been published demonstrating safety and efficacy in pediatric and adult patients at 24 weeks of treatment; CACT deficiency patients were excluded from this study due to the severity of the condition (Vockley et al. 2017).

Patients with CACT deficiency are at high risk for morbidity and mortality with each fasting period or illness. Despite maximizing supportive measures during a severe metabolic crisis, our patient's condition declined precipitously. Only after providing triheptanoin did cardiac function improve gradually but dramatically, with ejection fraction rising from 24.9 to 73.7%. With continuation of triheptanoin as a routine part of her nutritional management, her cardiac function remained preserved through the next 2 years of life. She even developed the ability to sit independently. Her ultimate death seemed linked to a primary respiratory event rather than a cardiac one. Given the paucity of clinical experience with triheptanoin use specifically in CACT deficiency, our report highlights the safe and efficacious use of triheptanoin in acute heart failure in this subset of patients. Triheptanoin may provide a therapeutic alternative that could potentially lead to improved outcomes for CACT deficiency patients.

Synopsis

This report details the safe use of triheptanoin to reverse cardiogenic shock in the case of a patient with carnitine-acylcarnitine translocase deficiency suffering severe metabolic crisis devolving into acute heart failure.

Compliance with Ethical Guidelines

As the submitting author, I confirm that all authors have adhered to strict ethical guidelines in the generation of this manuscript.

Contributor's Statement

Sidharth Mahapatra contributed to the conception and design of this case presentation, the literature search, drafting the initial manuscript, and revising and reviewing the manuscript.

Amitha Ananth, Nancy Baugh, and Mihaela Damian reviewed and revised the manuscript.

Mihaela Damian contributed to the conception and design of the case presentation and gathered the data to generate the tables and figure.

Gregory Enns contributed to the conception and design of the case presentation, and reviewed and revised the manuscript. He was a member of the UX007 data safety monitoring board.

All authors approved the final manuscript as submitted and agree to be accountable for all aspects of the work.

References

Bonnet D, Martin D, Pascale De L, Villain E, Jouvet P, Rabier D, Brivet M, Saudubray JM (1999) Arrhythmias and conduction defects as presenting symptoms of fatty acid oxidation disorders in children. Circulation 100:2248–2253

Eto K, Sakai N, Shimada S, Shioda M, Ishigaki K, Hamada Y, Shinpo M, Azuma J, Tominaga K, Shimojima K, Ozono K, Osawa M, Yamamoto T (2013) Microdeletions of 3p21.31 characterized by developmental delay, distinctive features, elevated serum creatine kinase levels, and white matter involvement. Am J Med Genet A 161a:3049–3056

Haldeman-Englert CR, Gai X, Perin JC, Ciano M, Halbach SS, Geiger EA, McDonald-McGinn DM, Hakonarson H, Zackai EH, Shaikh TH (2009) A 3.1-Mb microdeletion of 3p21.31 associated with cortical blindness, cleft lip, CNS abnormalities, and developmental delay. Eur J Med Genet 52:265–268

Hsu BY, Iacobazzi V, Wang Z, Harvie H, Chalmers RA, Saudubray JM, Palmieri F, Ganguly A, Stanley CA (2001) Aberrant mRNA splicing associated with coding region mutations in children with carnitine-acylcarnitine translocase deficiency. Mol Genet Metab 74:248–255

Pande SV, Murthy MS (1994) Carnitine-acylcarnitine translocase deficiency: implications in human pathology. Biochim Biophys Acta 1226:269–276

Roe CR, Brunengraber H (2015) Anaplerotic treatment of long-chain fat oxidation disorders with triheptanoin: review of 15 years experience. Mol Genet Metab 116:260–268

Roe CR, Mochel F (2006) Anaplerotic diet therapy in inherited metabolic disease: therapeutic potential. J Inherit Metab Dis 29:332–340

Roe CR, Sweetman L, Roe DS, David F, Brunengraber H (2002) Treatment of cardiomyopathy and rhabdomyolysis in long-chain fat oxidation disorders using an anaplerotic odd-chain triglyceride. J Clin Invest 110:259–269

Rubio-Gozalbo ME, Bakker JA, Waterham HR, Wanders RJ (2004) Carnitine-acylcarnitine translocase deficiency, clinical, biochemical and genetic aspects. Mol Asp Med 25:521–532

Spiekerkoetter U, Lindner M, Santer R, Grotzke M, Baumgartner MR, Boehles H, Das A, Haase C, Hennermann JB, Karall D, de Klerk H, Knerr I, Koch HG, Plecko B, Roschinger W, Schwab KO, Scheible D, Wijburg FA, Zschocke J, Mayatepek E, Wendel U (2009) Management and outcome in 75 individuals with long-chain fatty acid oxidation defects: results from a workshop. J Inherit Metab Dis 32:488–497

Stanley CA, Hale DE, Berry GT, Deleeuw S, Boxer J, Bonnefont JP (1992) Brief report: a deficiency of carnitine-acylcarnitine translocase in the inner mitochondrial membrane. N Engl J Med 327:19–23

Vitoria I, Martin-Hernandez E, Pena-Quintana L, Bueno M, Quijada-Fraile P, Dalmau J, Molina-Marrero S, Perez B, Merinero B (2015) Carnitine-acylcarnitine translocase deficiency: experience with four cases in Spain and review of the literature. JIMD Rep 20:11–20

Vockley J, Marsden D, McCracken E, DeWard S, Barone A, Hsu K, Kakkis E (2015) Long-term major clinical outcomes in patients with long chain fatty acid oxidation disorders before and after transition to triheptanoin treatment – a retrospective chart review. Mol Genet Metab 116:53–60

Vockley J, Charrow J, Ganesh J, Eswara M, Diaz GA, McCracken E, Conway R, Enns GM, Starr J, Wang R, Abdenur JE, Sanchez-de-Toledo J, Marsden DL (2016) Triheptanoin treatment in patients with pediatric cardiomyopathy associated with long chain-fatty acid oxidation disorders. Mol Genet Metab 119:223–231

Vockley J, Burton B, Berry GT, Longo N, Phillips J, Sanchez-Valle A, Tanpaiboon P, Grunewald S, Murphy E, Humphrey R, Mayhew J, Bowden A, Zhang L, Cataldo J, Marsden DL, Kakkis E (2017) UX007 for the treatment of long chain-fatty acid oxidation disorders: safety and efficacy in children and adults following 24 weeks of treatment. Mol Genet Metab 120(4):370–377

JIMD Reports
DOI 10.1007/8904_2017_44

RESEARCH REPORT

Glutaric Aciduria Type 1 and Acute Renal Failure: Case Report and Suggested Pathomechanisms

Marcel du Moulin · Bastian Thies · Martin Blohm ·
Jun Oh · Markus J. Kemper · René Santer ·
Chris Mühlhausen

Received: 18 May 2017 / Revised: 14 June 2017 / Accepted: 22 June 2017 / Published online: 12 July 2017
© SSIEM and Springer-Verlag Berlin Heidelberg 2017

Abstract Glutaric aciduria type 1 (GA1) is caused by deficiency of the mitochondrial matrix enzyme glutaryl-CoA dehydrogenase (GCDH), leading to accumulation of glutaric acid (GA) and 3-hydroxyglutaric acid (3OHGA) in tissues and body fluids. During catabolic crises, GA1 patients are prone to the development of striatal necrosis and a subsequent irreversible movement disorder during a time window of vulnerability in early infancy. Thus, GA1 had been considered a pure "cerebral organic aciduria" in the past. Single case reports have indicated the occurrence of acute renal dysfunction in children affected by GA1. In addition, growing evidence arises that GA1 patients may develop chronic renal failure during adulthood independent of the previous occurrence of encephalopathic crises. The underlying mechanisms are yet unknown. Here we report on a 3-year-old GA1 patient who died following the development of acute renal failure most likely due to haemolytic uraemic syndrome associated with a pneumococcal infection. We hypothesise that known GA1 pathomechanisms, namely the endothelial dysfunction mediated by 3OHGA, as well as the transporter mechanisms for the urinary excretion of GA and 3OHGA, are involved in the development of glomerular and tubular dysfunction, respectively, and may contribute to a pre-disposition of GA1 patients to renal disease. We recommend careful differential monitoring of glomerular and tubular renal function in GA1 patients.

Communicated by: Georg Hoffmann

M. du Moulin · B. Thies · M. Blohm · J. Oh · M.J. Kemper · R. Santer · C. Mühlhausen (✉)
University Children's Hospital, University Medical Center Hamburg-Eppendorf, Martinistrasse 52, Building O45,
20246 Hamburg, Germany
e-mail: muehlhausen@uke.de

Abbreviations

3OHGA	3-Hydroxyglutaric acid
E-IMD	European registry and network for intoxication-type metabolic diseases
GA	Glutaric acid
GA1	Glutaric aciduria type 1
GCDH	Glutaryl-CoA dehydrogenase
GFR	Glomerular filtration rate
HUS	Haemolytic uraemic syndrome
LDH	Lactate dehydrogenase
OAD	Organic aciduria

Introduction

Glutaric aciduria type 1 (GA1, OMIM 231670) is caused by the autosomal-recessively inherited deficiency of glutaryl-CoA dehydrogenase (GCDH, E.C. 1.3.8.6), a mitochondrial matrix enzyme involved in the degradation of lysine and tryptophan. Affected patients accumulate the pathologic metabolites glutaric acid (GA) and 3-hydroxyglutaric acid (3OHGA) and glutaryl-CoA, and are prone to encephalopathic crises during a time window of vulnerability up to 72 months of age, with subsequent irreversible movement disorder due to injury of striatal neurons (Goodman and Frerman 2001). Early diagnosis of the disease by newborn screening is essential to avoid irreversible neurological sequelae. Treatment includes presymptomatic implementation of a lysine-restricted diet, carnitine supplementation, and a sufficient emergency management to avoid catabolism (Boy et al. 2017). The impairment of mitochondrial energy production reported in various in vitro and in vivo models appears to play a role in the pathophysiology of GA1, although the pathomechanisms leading to neurodegeneration are not yet fully understood (Jafari et al. 2011; Lamp et al. 2011). Animal and cellular models have demonstrated that the blood–brain barrier shows only very limited permeability for GA and 3OHGA. Thus, when produced intracerebrally, these metabolites accumulate in the brain compartment (Keyser et al. 2008; Sauer et al. 2006). GA and 3OHGA are excreted into urine via active tubular transport processes (Mühlhausen et al. 2008).

The haemolytic uraemic syndrome (HUS) belongs to the thrombotic microangiopathies. It commonly occurs in children and presents primarily with renal failure, haemolytic anaemia and thrombocytopenia. The most abundant trigger is the Shiga toxin of enterohaemorrhagic *E. coli*. But also other causes, e.g. inborn deficiencies in the complement system, or invasive *Streptococcus pneumoniae* infections, have been reported (Noris et al. 2012).

Here, we report on a 3-year-old girl with GA1 who died from renal failure most likely caused by pneumococcus-associated HUS. We hypothesise that GA1 may have been a predisposing factor for the acute renal failure that complicated this patient's pneumococcal sepsis, in that GA1 may promote increased endothelial vulnerability and thus the development of HUS.

Case Presentation

The girl was the first child of healthy, consanguineous parents of Turkish descent. GA1 was diagnosed by newborn screening. Subsequently, analysis of organic acids in urine detected a "high excretor" status (GA 2,650 mmol/mol creatinine; 3OHGA 92 mmol/mol creatinine; Baric et al. 1999). Genetic analysis revealed the homozygous pathogenic variant p.Arg402Trp in the *GCDH* gene, and residual GCDH enzyme activity in fibroblasts was found to be absent. A lysine-restricted diet, carnitine supplementation and adequate emergency management were implemented according to current therapy guidelines (Boy et al. 2017). Until the age of 3 years, the clinical course was uneventful with normal psychomotor development, absence of encephalopathic crises and lack of any signs of a movement disorder.

During a holiday trip to Turkey at the age of 3 years and 3 months, the girl suffered from a febrile airway infection. She developed dyspnoea and refused to eat. Her condition rapidly deteriorated and the parents decided to return to Germany for medical treatment. The parents tried to apply maltodextrin solution for anabolisation, but the girl drank only small amounts. During the flight, her consciousness was reduced and she developed haematemesis.

On admission, the girl was somnolent, had fever and presented with tachypnoea. During the initial clinical examination, no signs of a movement disorder were observed. Severe metabolic acidosis was found (pH 7.19, bicarbonate 8.9 mmol/L, base excess −17.7 mmol/L, pCO$_2$ 23 mmHg) and metabolic emergency treatment was instituted including discontinuation of all protein intake and intravenous administration of high glucose-containing solution, insulin and carnitine. Due to persisting massive tachydyspnoea and increasing respiratory failure, intubation and mechanical ventilation were necessary. Inflammatory parameters were elevated (leukocytes 16.4/nL [normal 5.5–15.5], C-reactive protein 160 mg/L [normal <0.5], procalcitonin 45 µg/L [normal <0.5]), and a chest X-ray indicated pneumonia. *Streptococcus pneumoniae*, serotype 14, was isolated in her blood culture and tracheal aspirate. In tracheal aspirate, rhinovirus could also be detected. The girl was diagnosed with invasive septic infection with *Streptococcus pneumoniae* and received appropriate antibiotic treatment. Of note, the girl had timely received all standard vaccinations including a 13-valent pneumococcal conjugate vaccine covering serotype 14 but apparently had not developed an appropriate immunity for unknown reasons; there were no clinical or laboratory signs of immune deficiency (normal IgG, normal red blood count, no increased frequency of infections prior to the episode described here). However, a specific work-up for immune deficiency was not performed.

Furthermore, the girl suffered from acute renal failure (creatinine 1.68 mg/dL [normal 0.2–0.75], blood urea nitrogen 66 mg/dL [normal 5–17]). Renal ultrasound revealed bilateral swelling, cortical hyperechogenicity and subcortical hypoperfusion. She also had anaemia (haemoglobin 9.6 g/dL [normal 10.1–13.1]) and showed signs of haemolysis (LDH 1,892 U/L [normal 120–300], raised up to 2,837 U/L the following days). Creatine kinase was elevated on admission (827 U/L [normal <148]) but normalised within 2 days, indicating absence of rhabdomyolysis. Platelets were elevated on admission but fell to 40,000/µL (normal 150,000–500,000) on the second day. A blood smear showed schistocytes. This combination of acute renal failure, haemolytic anaemia and thrombocytopenia lead to the clinical diagnosis of atypical haemolytic uraemic syndrome (HUS) associated with pneumococcal disease. Unfortunately, the girl's condition did not allow for renal biopsy to confirm the diagnosis histologically. Analyses of urine revealed a pronounced glomerular and tubular proteinuria (albumin maximum 4,857 mg/g creatinine [normal <30]; alpha-1-microglobulin maximum 193 mg/g creatinine [normal <30]).

Due to a further decline of urine output and increasing renal retention parameters (creatinine maximum 2.99 mg/dL;

cystatine c maximum 3.19 mg/L [normal 0.53–0.95]; GFR calculated from cystatine c minimum 25 mL/min) peritoneal dialysis was started on day 3 of hospitalisation and had to be changed to haemodialysis on day 6. In addition, plasmapheresis was performed several times as an attempt to treat the HUS. Determination of acylcarnitines in dried blood spots during renal failure revealed an elevation of free carnitine (917 μmol/L [normal 10–70]) and all acylcarnitines, especially glutarylcarnitine (364 μmol/L [normal <0.4]). Determination of organic acids in urine showed a vastly elevated concentration of lactate (15,025 mmol/mol creatinine [normal <285]) and glutarate (4,839 mmol/mol creatinine [normal <5]), and a slight elevation of concentrations of citric acid cycle intermediates (succinate 203 mmol/mol creatinine [normal <79]; fumarate 34 mmol/mol creatinine [normal <10]) and ketones (2-hydroxybutyrate 271 mmol/mol creatinine [normal <5]; 3-hydroxybutyrate 135 mmol/mol creatinine [normal <11]). 3OHGA was not detectable in this sample. No clinical signs of a movement disorder were detected at any time; however, the validity of neurological exam was restricted due to sedation. The girl's condition did not permit an MRI scan, but on day 13 a cranial CT scan was performed to assess for brain abnormalities. This scan revealed enlarged Sylvian fissures (stable as compared to MRI findings at age 1 month); the basal ganglia did not show any abnormalities. Taken together, neither clinical nor radiographic signs of an encephalopathic crisis were detected.

The clinical course was further complicated by severe lactic acidosis. For a short period of time, reduction of glucose administration had a positive effect. However, lactate concentrations increased again and were persistently elevated above 30 mmol/L for several days, and were refractory to any therapeutic intervention. The girl died 22 days after admission due to multiple organ failure. Postmortem was declined by the parents.

Discussion

Here, we report on a patient with GA1 and acute renal failure most likely due to atypical HUS caused by invasive pneumococcal disease.

Renal involvement has not been considered to be part of the phenotypic spectrum of GA1 previously. However, it has been shown that 20–25% of adults with GA1 above the age of 20 years suffer from chronic renal failure (Kölker et al. 2015). In addition, there have been single reports about patients with GA1 and renal disease (Table 1). Pöge and colleagues described a patient with GA1 who first presented with neurologic symptoms in the neonatal period and developed nephrotic syndrome at the age of 12 weeks with glomerular damage, crescentic glomerulonephritis but

a normal tubular morphology (Pöge et al. 1997). In another report, a 6-year-old patient with GA1 was described suffering from acute renal failure requiring dialysis. Similar to our case, HUS had initially been suspected in this patient because of accompanying anaemia and thrombocytopenia. However, kidney biopsy in this patient revealed significant acute tubular damage with distended tubules, damaged epithelial cells and loss of the brush border membrane, while the glomeruli were morphologically intact (Pode-Shakked et al. 2014). Interestingly, the tubular morphology reported in this case resembles the renal alterations observed in a mouse model of GA1 during induced metabolic crises (Thies et al. 2013). In the latter study, during metabolic crises induced by the administration of a high protein diet, Gcdh-deficient mice showed an acute tubular damage with functional tubulopathy, a thinning of brush border membranes in renal proximal tubule cells and an altered mitochondrial morphology with enlargement of mitochondria and a reduction in electron density.

In the patient reported here, from the clinical point of view the acute renal failure had been attributed to atypical HUS caused by proven pneumococcal sepsis. Due to the lack of renal histology, however, it cannot be excluded that our patient alternatively or in addition suffered from acute tubular damage as reported earlier in a patient with initial suspicion of HUS (Pode-Shakked et al. 2014), as indicated by the elevated urinary excretion of the tubulopathy marker alpha-1-microglobulin in our patient.

Taken together, it cannot be proven whether the metabolic (GA1) and renal (HUS) diseases in our patient were inter-related or rather independent events. However, the increasing evidence that in GA1 patients chronic renal failure develops over time (Kölker et al. 2015), and single cases of GA1 patients with acute renal diseases as presented here, suggest that the metabolic alterations in GA1 may display a pre-disposing factor for the development of acute and/or chronic renal disease.

Various pathomechanisms may be involved in renal disease in GA1 patients:

1. The pathophysiology of both GA1 and HUS involves microangiopathy: HUS is associated with thrombotic microangiopathy of glomerular endothelium (Noris et al. 2012), whereas in the presence of the GA1-specific metabolite 3OHGA the endothelial integrity was impaired in in vitro and in vivo models of endothelial barriers (Mühlhausen et al. 2006). The impaired endothelial integrity due to the disease-specific metabolites may pre-dispose GA1 patients to HUS-specific microangiopathy as an add-on pathogenic event, thus making GA1 patients more prone to the development of HUS.

Table 1 Functional and histologic renal alterations in GA1 patients

Model	Renal dysfunction	Glomerular histology	Tubular histology	Reference
Case report	Nephrotic syndrome	Crescentic glomerulonephritis: shrinking of glomerular tufts, increased mesangial matrix, extracapillary epithelial proliferations, formation of larger epithelial crescents	Normal	Pöge et al. (1997)
GA1 mouse model	Tubulopathy	Normal	Acute tubular damage: thinned bush border membrane, altered mitochondrial morphology with enlargement and reduced electron density	Thies et al. (2013)
Case report	Acute renal failure, proteinuria, suspected HUS	Normal	Acute tubular necrosis: tubular damage with distended tubules, damaged epithelial cells, loss of brush border, debris in the tubular lumen, interstitial oedema	Pode-Shakked et al. (2014)
E-IMD study population (GA1, $n = 150$; 14% of OAD cohort adult patients)	Chronic renal failure in 25% of adult patients >20 years of age	Not reported	Not reported	Kölker et al. (2015)
Case report	Acute renal failure, suspected HUS; proteinuria (albumin, alpha-1-microglobulin)	Not done	Not done	This report

2. Renal proximal tubule cells express various transporters that mediate the urinary excretion of GA and 3OHGA (Hagos et al. 2008; Mühlhausen et al. 2008; Stellmer et al. 2007); the expression of these transporters is altered during induced metabolic crises in a GA1 mouse model, which may result in an intracellular accumulation of GA and 3OHGA in renal proximal tubule cells, contributing to an impairment of mitochondrial energy production in these cells (Thies et al. 2013). Thus, a severely catabolising condition such as an invasive pneumococcal disease may lead to metabolic decompensation and an increase of GA and 3OHGA concentrations in proximal tubule cells. This may promote a continuously progressive renal proximal tubule dysfunction, eventually leading to acute tubular damage and renal failure. In addition, non-acute but chronic exposure of renal proximal tubule cells to GA and 3OHGA may account for the chronic development of a tubular disease and eventually chronic renal failure as reported in adult GA1 patients. The potential role of renal proximal tubule cells in the development of GA1-associated renal disease is in line with recent observations of a high renal GCDH expression specifically in proximal tubule cells (Braissant et al. 2017).

Conclusion

This case report adds to the growing evidence of acute and chronic renal disease in GA1 triggered by acute catabolic events or developing over time, respectively. Further research is necessary to unravel the underlying mechanisms. With regard to patient care, we consider it important to carefully monitor glomerular as well as tubular function in GA1 patients to detect a potential impairment of renal function as early as possible.

Synopsis

We report on a 3-year-old GA1 patient with acute renal failure most likely due to haemolytic uraemic syndrome associated with a pneumococcal infection. Endothelial dysfunction and renal proximal tubule accumulation of

GA1 metabolites may contribute to acute and chronic glomerular and tubular dysfunction in GA1 patients.

Compliance with Ethics Guidelines

Conflict of Interest Statement

Marcel du Moulin, Bastian Thies, Martin Blohm, Jun Oh, Markus J. Kemper, René Santer and Chris Mühlhausen declare that they have no conflict of interest.

Informed Consent

The study does not contain any identifying information about patients.

This chapter does not contain any studies with human or animal subjects performed by any of the authors.

Details of the Contributions of Individual Authors

Marcel du Moulin: Dr. du Moulin cared for the patient, performed collection and analyses of the data, drafted and critically reviewed the manuscript and approved the final manuscript as submitted.

Bastian Thies: Dr. Thies cared for the patient, performed collection and analyses of the data, drafted and critically reviewed the manuscript and approved the final manuscript as submitted.

Martin Blohm: Dr. Blohm cared for the patient, especially with regard to the intensive care management, carried out critical discussions regarding the pathophysiology of the patient, collected and analysed the data, reviewed and revised the manuscript and approved the final manuscript as submitted.

Jun Oh: Dr. Oh carried out and critically discussed the nephrologic treatment of the patient (dialysis procedures), collected and critically discussed the data, reviewed and revised the manuscript and approved the final manuscript as submitted.

Markus J. Kemper: Dr. Kemper carried out and critically discussed the nephrologic treatment of the patient (dialysis procedures), collected and critically discussed the data, reviewed and revised the manuscript and approved the final manuscript as submitted.

René Santer: Dr. Santer carried out and critically discussed the metabolic treatment of the patient, critically analysed and reviewed the collected data, drafted, critically reviewed and revised the manuscript and approved the final manuscript as submitted.

Chris Mühlhausen: Dr. Mühlhausen carried out, critically discussed and reviewed the metabolic treatment of the patient, designed the data collection instruments, coordinated and supervised data collection and analyses, drafted and critically reviewed the manuscript and approved the final manuscript as submitted.

References

Baric I, Wagner L, Feyh P, Liesert M, Buckel W, Hoffmann GF (1999) Sensitivity and specificity of free and total glutaric acid and 3-hydroxyglutaric acid measurements by stable-isotope dilution assays for the diagnosis of glutaric aciduria type I. J Inherit Metab Dis 22:867–882

Boy N, Mühlhausen C, Maier EM et al (2017) Proposed recommendations for diagnosing and managing individuals with glutaric aciduria type I: second revision. J Inherit Metab Dis 40:75–101

Braissant O, Jafari P, Remacle N, Cudré-Cung H-P, do Vale Pereira S, Ballhausen D (2017) Immunolocalization of glutaryl-CoA dehydrogenase (GCDH) in adult and embryonic rat brain and peripheral tissues. Neuroscience 343:355–363

Goodman SI, Frerman FE (2001) Organic acidemias due to defects in lysine oxidation: 2-ketoadipic acidemia and glutaric acidemia. In: Scriver CR, Beaudet AL, Sly WS et al (eds) The metabolic and molecular bases of inherited disease. McGraw-Hill, New York, pp 2195–2204

Hagos Y, Krick W, Braulke T, Mühlhausen C, Burckhardt G, Burckhardt BC (2008) Organic anion transporters OAT1 and OAT4 mediate the high affinity transport of glutarate derivatives accumulating in patients with glutaric acidurias. Pflugers Arch 457:223–231

Jafari P, Braissant O, Bonafé L, Ballhausen D (2011) The unsolved puzzle of neuropathogenesis in glutaric aciduria type I. Mol Genet Metab 104:425–437

Keyser B, Glatzel M, Stellmer F et al (2008) Transport and distribution of 3-hydroxyglutaric acid before and during induced encephalopathic crises in a mouse model of glutaric aciduria type 1. Biochim Biophys Acta 1782:385–390

Kölker S, Valayannopoulos V, Burlina AB et al (2015) The phenotypic spectrum of organic acidurias and urea cycle disorders. Part 2: The evolving clinical phenotype. J Inherit Metab Dis 38:1059–1074

Lamp J, Keyser B, Koeller DM, Ullrich K, Braulke T, Mühlhausen C (2011) Glutaric aciduria type 1 metabolites impair the succinate transport from astrocytic to neuronal cells. J Biol Chem 286:17777–17784

Mühlhausen C, Ott N, Chalajour F et al (2006) Endothelial effects of 3-hydroxyglutaric acid: implications for glutaric aciduria type I. Pediatr Res 59:196–202

Mühlhausen C, Burckhardt BC, Hagos Y et al (2008) Membrane translocation of glutaric acid and its derivatives. J Inherit Metab Dis 31:188–193

Noris M, Mescia F, Remuzzi G (2012) STEC-HUS, atypical HUS and TTP are all diseases of complement activation. Nat Rev Nephrol 8:622–633

Pode-Shakked B, Marek-Yagel D, Rubinshtein M et al (2014) Glutaric aciduria type I and acute renal failure – coincidence or causality? Mol Genet Metab Rep 1:170–175

Pöge AP, Autschbach F, Korall H, Trefz FK, Mayatepek E (1997) Early clinical manifestation of glutaric aciduria type I and nephrotic syndrome during the first months of life. Acta Paediatr 86:1144–1147

Sauer SW, Okun JG, Fricker G et al (2006) Intracerebral accumulation of glutaric and 3-hydroxyglutaric acids secondary to limited flux across the blood-brain barrier constitute a biochemical risk factor for neurodegeneration in glutaryl-CoA dehydrogenase deficiency. J Neurochem 97:899–910

Stellmer F, Keyser B, Burckhardt BC et al (2007) 3-Hydroxyglutaric acid is transported via the sodium-dependent dicarboxylate transporter NaDC3. J Mol Med 85:763–770

Thies B, Meyer-Schwesinger C, Lamp J et al (2013) Acute renal proximal tubule alterations during induced metabolic crises in a mouse model of glutaric aciduria type 1. Biochim Biophys Acta 1832:1463–1472

JIMD Reports
DOI 10.1007/8904_2017_43

RESEARCH REPORT

Cardiovascular Histopathology of a 11-Year Old with Mucopolysaccharidosis VII Demonstrates Fibrosis, Macrophage Infiltration, and Arterial Luminal Stenosis

Valerie Lew · Louis Pena · Robert Edwards · Raymond Y. Wang

Received: 05 April 2017 / Revised: 19 June 2017 / Accepted: 22 June 2017 / Published online: 13 July 2017
© SSIEM and Springer-Verlag Berlin Heidelberg 2017

Abstract Mucopolysaccharidosis type VII (MPS VII) is caused by β-glucuronidase deficiency, resulting in lysosomal accumulation of glycosaminoglycans (GAGs) and multisystemic disease. We present cardiovascular gross and histopathology findings from a 11-year-old MPS VII male, who expired after developing ventricular fibrillation following anesthesia induction. Gross anatomic observations were made at autopsy; postmortem formalin-fixed paraffin-embedded samples of the carotid artery, aorta, myocardium, and valves were sectioned and stained with hematoxylin-eosin, Verhoeff-Van Gieson, CD68, and trichrome stains. Gross heart findings include an enlarged, dilated heart, mitral valve prolapse with thick, shortened chordae tendinae, and thickened aortic valve cusps. The aorta contained raised intimal plaques mimicking conventional atherosclerosis. Cardiac myocytes included hypertrophic nuclei, subendocardial fibrosis, and increased interfascicular collagen. Coronary lumens were 40–70% stenosed by fibrointimal hyperplasia containing storage material-laden cells, CD68[+] macrophages, and fragmented elastin laminae. Similar findings were visualized in aortic intimal plaques. We confirm that arterial plaques, elastin fragmentation, and activated CD68[+] macrophage infiltration occur in human MPS VII, consistent with previously observed findings in murine and canine MPS VII. We also confirm ultrasonographically observed carotid intimal-medial thickening is an in vivo correlate of histopathologic vascular fibrointimal hyperplasia. MPS VII patients should be regularly monitored for cardiac disease, with methods such as Holter monitors and stress testing; MPS VII-directed treatments should effectively address cardiovascular disease.

Communicated by: Frits Wijburg

V. Lew
UC Riverside School of Medicine, Riverside, CA 92521, USA

L. Pena
Los Angeles County Department of Medical Examiner-Coroner, Los Angeles, CA 90033, USA

L. Pena
Hidalgo Medical Services, Lordsburg, NM 88045, USA

R. Edwards
Department of Pathology & Lab Medicine, University of California, Irvine School of Medicine, Orange, CA 92868, USA

R.Y. Wang
Department of Pediatrics, University of California, Irvine School of Medicine, Orange, CA 92868, USA

R.Y. Wang (✉)
Division of Metabolic Disorders, Children's Hospital of Orange County, Orange, CA 92868, USA
e-mail: rawang@choc.org

Introduction

The mucopolysaccharidoses (MPSs) are inherited lysosomal storage diseases caused by deficiencies of enzymes involved in catabolism of glycosaminoglycans (GAGs). MPS type VII is caused by a deficiency of the lysosomal enzyme β-glucuronidase, which results in systemic accumulation of GAGs, specifically chondroitin sulfate (CS), dermatan sulfate (DS), and heparan sulfate (HS). Due to the ubiquitous nature of these GAGs, clinical manifestations of MPS VII include varying degrees of nonimmune hydrops fetalis, cognitive impairment, corneal clouding, airway obstruction, hepatosplenomegaly, orthopedic disease, and cardiovascular disease (Montaño et al. 2016). Even amongst MPSs, MPS VII is a rare condition, affecting 1 in every 345,000–2,000,000 live births (Muenzer 2011).

Sudden death has been described in two older patients, and corresponding reports of cardiovascular histopathology are also minimal (Vogler et al. 1994; Metcalf et al. 2010; Bigg et al. 2013; Gniadek et al. 2015). We describe the cardiovascular histopathology findings in a 11-year-old boy with MPS VII who died after sustaining ventricular tachycardia during a dental procedure under anesthesia, and relate the findings to findings in animal models of MPS VII that may shed light upon pathogenesis of MPS-associated cardiovascular disease. An up to date summary compiling hypothesis from literature on MPS VII pathogenesis is included to demonstrate the limited research.

Materials and Methods

Human Subjects

Consent for retrospective chart review and postmortem tissue donation was obtained from parents (Children's Hospital of Orange County IRB #100109, approved 12 Apr 2010).

Pathology

Tissue samples of the heart, ascending and descending aorta, rib cartilage, and spinal cord were frozen at $-80°C$. Additional formalin-fixed, paraffin embedded tissue samples from the Los Angeles County Coroners' office were sectioned and stained.

Histopathology

Tissue samples frozen in OCT were sectioned on a Leica CM3050 cryostat and stained with hematoxylin and eosin. Cytochemical stains for elastic fibers (Verhoeff-Van Gieson stain), glycosaminoglycan (Alcian Blue stain pH 2.5), collagen (Mallory Trichrome stain), and immunohistochemical stains for anti-human CD68 were performed on a Ventana Benchmark Ultra autostainer. Immunohistochemical staining was developed with peroxidase-based detection.

Results

Case Report

This patient was briefly reported in Montaño et al. (2016) as patient 12 (Montaño et al. 2016). His prenatal history was significant for hydrops fetalis noted at 8 months' gestation, and he was born at 38 weeks' gestational age due to pregnancy-induced hypertension and maternal protein-uria. Neonatal respiratory failure necessitated intubation and mechanical ventilation until the hydrops resolved. Organomegaly, thrombocytopenia, conjugated hyperbilirubinemia, and bilateral inguinal hernias were also present in the neonatal period leading to diagnosis of MPS VII.

He was lost to follow-up until 7 years of age, when he presented for medical attention for his MPS due to progressive behavioral difficulties and painful bilateral hip dysplasia. He had recurrent otitis media requiring ear tube implantation, hepatosplenomegaly, kyphoscoliosis, and obstructive sleep apnea. Urinary GAGs were quantitatively elevated at 32.9 mg/mmol creatinine (reference range <12 mg/mmol creatinine) and qualitatively demonstrated excess CS, DS, and HS. Molecular sequencing of the β-glucuronidase gene *GUSB* identified compound heterozygous, previously unreported c.295G>A/c.866G>A (p. V99M/W289X) variants.

The patient had quarterly electrocardiograms, echocardiograms, and cardiology evaluations. His initial echocardiogram at age 7.5 years showed mild aortic insufficiency, mild-moderate mitral insufficiency, mild left ventricular (LV) dilation, and normal fractional shortening (FS) of 35%. He was placed on enalapril due to the mitral insufficiency. Over the next 4 years, serial echocardiograms identified thickening of the mitral and aortic valves, mild mitral valve prolapse, mildly impaired LV relaxation, then mild-moderate diminished LV systolic function with an ejection fraction of 49% (reference range, >58%). At age 8.8 years, carotid ultrasonography identified greatly increased carotid intima media thickness (cIMT) of 0.50 mm on the right and 0.53 mm on the left compared to controls (mean control cIMT 0.48 mm, standard deviation 0.034 cm) (Wang et al. 2011).

His behavioral difficulties made it difficult to adequately keep up with his dental care, and the patient was therefore admitted for oral cleaning under anesthesia. He was administered Sevoflurane, and shortly after, he spontaneously developed ventricular tachycardia that rapidly degenerated to ventricular fibrillation. Efforts to resuscitate the patient were unsuccessful. Further pathology investigation identified primary cardiac etiology as cause of death.

Histopathology

Parental consent was given for postmortem studies. Weighing 275 g, more than twice the mean for age (122 g) (Hamill et al. 1979), the heart and especially the left ventricle were grossly enlarged and dilated. The mitral valve revealed ballooning of the leaflets with thick and shortened chordae tendinae. The aortic valve cusps were also thickened. Raised intimal plaques were visualized throughout the ascending and descending aorta. Noncardiac gross findings included cerebral edema, mucous plugging of the conducting airways of the lung, and hepatospleno-megaly.

Microscopically, the sinoatrial, atrioventricular nodes, and conduction system were unremarkable. However, the myocardium contained hypertrophic cardiomyocytes with characteristic "boxcar" nuclei, prominent subendocardial fibrosis, and increased interfascicular collagen, consistent with chronic ischemic heart disease (Geer et al. 1980). Severe myxomatous degeneration (red arrowheads, Fig. 1a–c) and fibrosis (white arrowheads, Fig. 1b) were visualized in the mitral and aortic valves. The surface of the mitral valve was rich with numerous CD68$^+$ macrophages, which are usually not present in normal mitral valves (Fig. 1c: brown-stained cells marked with m).

Coronary lumens were 40–70% stenosed by intimal hyperplasia (Fig. 2a, b) that was shown to be composed of glycosaminoglycan-rich matrix (Fig. 2c: blue periodic acid-Schiff staining marked with g), storage-laden cells (Fig. 2d, examples marked with red arrowheads), fibrosis (Fig. 2d: blue Trichrome staining), fragmented elastin laminae (Fig. 2e: white arrowheads), and CD68$^+$ macrophages (Fig. 2g: brown-stained cells marked with m). None of the macrophages demonstrated lipid vacuole-laden cytoplasm and the hyperplastic regions showed no cholesterol-clefting. These findings are in dual contrast to normal arterial media, which has continuous sheets of elastin fibers and no macrophage infiltration, as well as to atherosclerotic plaques, which demonstrate "foamy" lipid-laden macrophages and cholesterol clefting (Miller 2014). Similar findings were seen focally in the aortic intimal plaques (Fig. 2e, f, h), though elastin fragmentation was less prominent compared to the coronary arteries.

Discussion

Cardiomyopathy and cardiac valve disease are very common manifestations of MPS VII, and frequently account for mortality in affected patients (Montaño et al. 2016). However, the pathogenesis of MPS VII cardiac disease is poorly understood due to scarce reports of human postmortem analyses. Of known histopathology reports of MPS VII patients (summarized in Table 1), most are in infants or fetal losses and very few focus upon the cardiovascular system. A MPS VII male who died suddenly at age 19 years demonstrated cardiac enlargement, thickening and calcification of the mitral and aortic valves, and plaques of the thoracic aorta and left anterior descending artery (Vogler et al. 1994). The aorta, which demonstrated cells distended with abundant storage material, was subsequently shown to have a large amount of elastin fragmentation (Metcalf et al. 2010). Cardiovascular pathology in a 28-year-old MPS VII patient who died in his sleep identified cardiac enlargement; myocardial interstitial fibrosis; pan-valvular thickening, fibrosis, and calcification; concentric narrowing of all coronary arteries with increased extracellular matrix, numerous CD68$^+$ macrophages, and mesenchymal cells distended by storage material (Gniadek et al. 2015). There was intimal-medial thickening of the aorta with disruption of the elastin laminae and scattered CD68$^+$ macrophages within.

Our patient demonstrated similar findings of cardiac enlargement and dilatation, subendocardial and interfascicular fibrosis, valve thickening, coronary artery stenosis and aortic plaques both demonstrating prominent intimal-medial hyperplasia, cellular GAG accumulation, CD68$^+$ macrophages, and fragmentation of the elastin laminae. Strikingly, these abnormalities were present at 11 years of age, indicating significant progression of MPS VII cardiovascular disease long before patients reach adulthood. The additional finding of carotid artery intimal-medial hyperplasia confirms the utility of carotid ultrasonography in identifying MPS-related cardiovascular disease in vivo. The pathologic findings (subendocardial myocardial fibrosis, dilated/hypertrophic cardiomyopathy, and anesthesia-induced hemodynamic changes) may all be manifestations

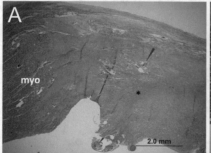
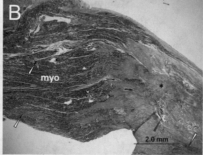
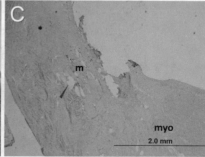

Fig. 1 Mitral valve and myocardial histopathology with (**a**) hematoxylin-eosin, (**b**) trichome stain, and (**c**) CD68 immunohistochemistry. Labels: *myo* myocardium, *asterisk* mitral valve, *m* macrophages. Myxomatous degeneration (*red arrowheads*), myocardial and valvular fibrosis (*white arrowheads*), and macrophage infiltration into valve parenchyma (*brown-stained cells*) are noted

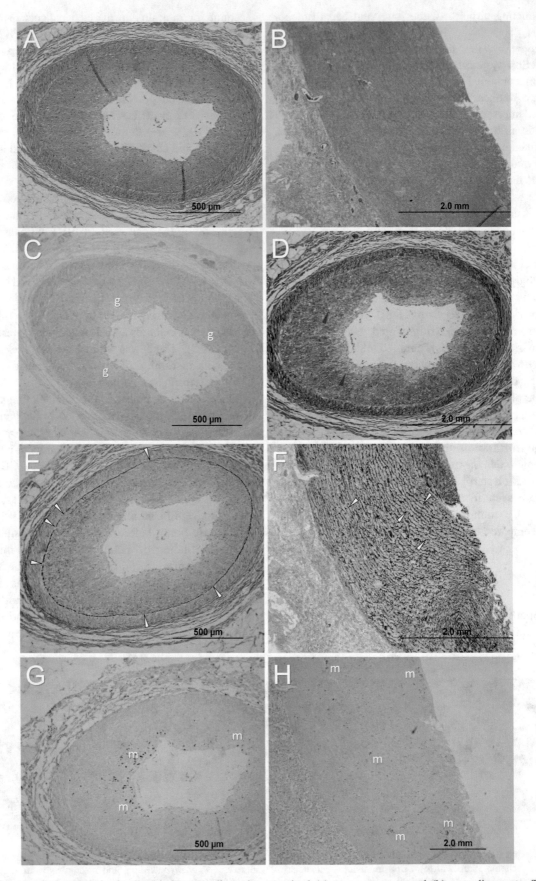

Fig. 2 Prominent luminal stenosis is visualized in hematoxylin-eosin   stained (**a**) coronary artery and (**b**) ascending aorta. The stenosing

of longstanding, ongoing ischemic heart disease and have contributed to the patient's fatal dysrhythmia (Toda et al. 2001).

While MPS VII cardiovascular lysosomal storage begins prenatally, the progression and pathogenesis of cardiomyopathy, valvular dysfunction, vascular intimal-medial hyperplasia, and elastin fragmentation are being elucidated (Irani et al. 1983; Molyneux et al. 1997; Geipel et al. 2002; Venkat-Raman et al. 2006; Delbecque et al. 2009). The canine model of MPS VII, which has a severe, rapidly progressive phenotype, shows mitral and aortic valve thickening as early as 0.3 years (Sammarco et al. 2000), and demonstrates similar cardiovascular histopathology (Muenzer 2011). MPS VII canine aortas also demonstrate reduced elastin content, increased protease expression and enzymatic activity, coupled with the abundance of activated macrophages and increased expression of immune sensing receptors (toll-like receptor 4) and proinflammatory cytokines (TNFα). Findings implicating GAG-induced inflammation in MPS I canine cardiovascular disease are highly suggestive of a similar mechanism taking place in MPS VII (Khalid et al. 2016). The finding of CD68[+] macrophages, which promote inflammation, within valve tissue and infiltrating arterial parenchyma in this patient lend credence to this hypothesis. Additional functional or expression studies are needed to confirm this hypothesis, highlighting the importance of postmortem tissue collection to understand pathophysiology of MPS VII disease.

Acknowledgments   The authors are grateful to the patient's parents for consenting to autopsy, and to Long Beach Memorial Hospital for obtaining autopsy consent. The authors are also grateful to the Los Angeles County Coroner's Office (Dan Anderson, Dr. Jason Tovar, Dr. Christopher Rogers, and Dr. Kevin Miller), and to Dr. Lisa Shane of Long Beach Miller Children's Hospital, for their efforts to make this publication possible. RYW is supported by the CHOC Children's Specialists Tithe Grant and the Brian and Caris Chan Family Foundation. The findings and conclusions in this chapter are those of the authors, and do not necessarily represent the official position of the County of Los Angeles or the Los Angeles County Department of the Medical Examiner-Coroner.

Synopsis

Significant cardiovascular disease (arterial fibrointimal stenosis, hypertrophic cardiomyopathy, valvular and myocardial fibrosis, and life-threatening dysrhythmias) was observed in a 11-year-old with mucopolysaccharidosis type VII; these findings indicate the importance of regular cardiology monitoring for MPS VII patients starting in early childhood.

Details of the Contributions of Individual Authors

- V.L. and R.Y.W. designed outline for manuscript as well as the figures
- L.P. performed postmortem
- L.P. and R.E. performed histopathology and interpretations
- V.L., L.P., R.E., and R.Y.W. wrote the manuscript

Name of the Corresponding Author

Raymond Y. Wang.

Competing Interest Statement

V.L., L.P., and R.E. have no conflicts of interest to declare. R.Y.W. is a study site principal investigator for a phase III study of recombinant human beta-glucuronidase for mucopolysaccharidosis type VII sponsored by Ultragenyx Pharmaceutical.

Details of Funding

This study was supported by CHOC Children's Specialists (V.L. and R.Y.W.), The Brian and Caris Chan Family Foundation (R.Y.W.), and The University of California-Riverside School of Medicine (V.L.).

Details of Ethics Approval

This report was conducted under the auspices of Children's Hospital of Orange County IRB #100109, approved 12 Apr 2010, renewed 17 Nov 2016.

A Patient Consent Statement

Consent for retrospective chart review and post mortem tissue donation was obtained from parents and is available for review upon request.

Fig. 2 (continued) lesions are composed of (**c**) glycosaminoglycans, as visualized by periodic acid-Schiff staining and denoted by *g*, (**d**) collagen fibrosis, and storage-containing "clear cells" (*red arrowheads*) as visualized by trichome staining. Elastin fragmentation (*white arrowheads*) was more notable in (**e**) the coronary artery than the (**f**) aorta. Macrophages, the CD68 (*brown*) staining cells marked with *m*, were also abundant within the lesions of (**g**) the coronary artery and (**h**) aorta but devoid of lipid-laden vacuoles

Table 1 Summary of the gross anatomy and histopathology findings of mucopolysaccharidosis type VII patients in the literature, including this report

MPS VII patient age of death (reference(s))	11 years (this report)	19 years (Vogler et al. 1994; Metcalf et al. 2010; Bigg et al. 2013)	28 years (Gniadek et al. 2015)	28 min (gest age unknown) (Irani et al. 1983)	Stillborn (32 weeks' gest) (Molyneux et al. 1997)	6 days (33 weeks' gest) (Geipel et al. 2002)	Fetal death (16 weeks' gest) (Venkat-Raman et al. 2006)	Termination (25 weeks' gest) (Delbecque et al. 2009)
Cardiac size	Enlarged	Slightly enlarged	Enlarged	n.m.	Dilatation	Hypertrophic	Normal	n.m.
Cardiac weight	275 g (nL 122 g)	400 g	484 g (nL 182–390 g)	n.m.	n.m.	n.m.	n.m.	n.m.
Mitral valve findings	Thick Fibrotic Myxomatous CD68+ cell infiltrate	Thick Calcified GAG storage Reduced collagen Neovascularized	Thick Fibrotic Nodular	n.m.	n.m.	n.m.	n.m.	n.m.
Aortic valve findings	Thick Fibrotic Myxomatous	Thick Nodular Calcified	Thick Nodular	n.m.	n.m.	n.m.	n.m.	n.m.
Coronary artery findings	Concentric narrowing Intimal thickening 40–70% stenosis CD68+ cell infiltrate	Eccentric narrowing 95% stenosis (left anterior descending)	Concentric narrowing Intimal thickening 75% stenosis (left anterior descending) 50–75% stenosis (circumflex) 75% stenosis (right coronary) CD68+ cell infiltrate	n.m.	n.m.	n.m.	n.m.	n.m.
Aortic findings	Visible plaque Intimal hyperplasia Elastin fragmentation CD68+ cells in plaque GAG accumulation	Visible plaques Elastin fragmentation Medial cells distended by storage Aortic dilatation	Visible thickening Intimal hyperplasia Elastin fragmentation CD68+ cells in plaque	n.m.	n.m.	n.m.	n.m.	Vacuolated aortic endothelium
Myocardium findings	Subendocardial fibrosis (prominent) Increased collagen, interfascicular Myocyte hypertrophy	n.m.	Thick myocardium Myocardial fibroelastosis Patchy interstitial fibrosis	n.m.	Vacuolated foamy myocardial cells	Vacuolated lysosomal overloading of myocytes	Normal microscopic exam of heart	n.m.
Other notes	Death from ventricular tachycardia Unremarkable SA/AV nodes	Death in sleep (aspiration vs. arrhythmia)	Death in sleep	Fetal hydrops GAG storage in cardiac capillary endothelium	Fetal hydrops	Fetal hydrops	Fetal hydrops	Fetal hydrops Vacuolated cardiac endothelium

Documentation of Approval from the Institutional Committee for Care and Use of Laboratory Animals (or Comparable Committee)

Not applicable (no animal studies).

References

Bigg PW, Baldo G, Sleeper MM, O'Donnell PA, Bai H, Rokkam VR, Liu Y, Wu S, Giugliani R, Casal ML, Haskins ME, Ponder KP (2013) Pathogenesis of mitral valve disease in mucopolysaccharidosis VII dogs. Mol Genet Metab 110:319–328

Delbecque K, Gaillez S, Schaaps JP (2009) Histopathological diagnosis of a type vii mucopolysaccharidosis after pregnancy termination. Fetal Pediatr Pathol 28(1):1–8

Geer JC, Crago CA, Little WC, Gardner LL, Bishop SP (1980) Subendocardial ischemic myocardial lesions associated with severe coronary atherosclerosis. Am J Pathol 98(3):663–680

Geipel A, Berg C, Germer U, Krapp M, Kohl M, Gembruch U (2002) Mucopolysaccharidosis VII (Sly disease) as a cause of increased nuchal translucency and non-immune fetal hydrops: study of a family and technical approach to prenatal diagnosis in early and late pregnancy. Prenat Diagn 22(6):493–495

Gniadek TJ, Singer N, Barker NJ, Spevak PJ, Crain BJ, Valle D, Halushka MK (2015) Cardiovascular pathologies in mucopolysaccharidosis type VII (Sly syndrome). Cardiovasc Pathol 24 (5):322–326

Hamill PV, Drizd TA, Johnson CL, Reed RB, Roche AF, Moore WM (1979) Physical growth: National Center for Health Statistics Percentiles. Am J Clin Nutr 32(3):607–629

Irani D, Kim HS, El-Hibri H, Dutton RV, Beaudet A, Armstrong D (1983) Postmortem observations on beta-glucuronidase deficiency presenting as hydrops fetalis. Ann Neurol 14(4):486–490

Khalid O, Vera MU, Gordts PL, Ellinwood NM, Schwartz PH, Dickson PI, Esko JD, Wang RY (2016) Immune-mediated inflammation may contribute to the pathogenesis of cardiovascular disease in mucopolysaccharidosis type I. PLoS One 11(3): e0150850

Metcalf JA, Linders B, Wu S, Bigg P, O'Donnell P, Sleeper MM, Whyte MP, Haskins M, Ponder KP (2010) Upregulation of elastase activity in aorta in mucopolysaccharidosis I and VII dogs may be due to increased cytokine expression. Mol Genet Metab 99(4):396–407

Miller DV (2014) Other pediatric cardiac conditions. In: Collins KA, Byard RW (eds) Forensic pathology of infancy and childhood. Springer, New York, pp 943–972

Molyneux AJ, Blair E, Coleman N, Daish P (1997) Mucopolysaccharidosis type VII associated with hydrops fetalis: histopathological and ultrastructural features with genetic implications. J Clin Pathol 50(3):252–254

Montaño AM, Lock-Hock N, Steiner RD, Graham BH, Szlago M, Greenstein R, Pineda M, Gonzalez-Meneses A, Coker M, Bartholomew D, Sands MS, Wang R, Giugliani R, Macaya A, Ketko AK, Ezgu F, Tanaka A, Arash L, Beck M, Falk RE, Bhattacharya K, Franco J, White KK, Mitchel GA, Cimbalistiene L, Holtz M, Sly WS (2016) Clinical course of sly syndrome (mucopolysaccharidosis type VII). J Med Genet 53(6):403–418

Muenzer J (2011) Overview of the mucopolysaccharidoses. Rheumatology 50(Suppl 5):v4–v12

Sammarco C, Weil M, Just C, Weimelt S, Hasson C, O'Malley T, Evans SM, Wang P, Casal ML, Wolfe J, Haskins M (2000) Effects of bone marrow transplantation on the cardiovascular abnormalities in canine mucopolysaccharidosis VII. Bone Marrow Transplant 25(12):1289–1297

Toda Y, Takeuchi M, Morita K, Iwasaki T, Oe K, Yokoyama M, Hirakawa M (2001) Complete heart block during anesthetic management in a patient with mucopolysaccharidosis type VII. Anesthesiology 95:1035–1037

Venkat-Raman N, Sebire NJ, Murphy KW (2006) Recurrent fetal hydrops due to mucopolysaccharidoses type VII. Fetal Diagn Ther 21(3):250–254

Vogler C, Levy B, Kyle JW, Sly WS, Williamson J, Whyte MP (1994) Mucopolysaccharidosis VII: postmortem biochemical and pathological findings in a young adult with beta-glucuronidase deficiency. Mod Pathol 7(1):132–137

Wang RY, Covault KK, Halcrow EM, Gardner AJ, Cao X, Newcomb RL, Dauben RD, Chang AC (2011) Carotid intima-media thickness is increased in patients with mucopolysaccharidoses. Mol Genet Metab 104(4):592–596

JIMD Reports
DOI 10.1007/8904_2017_42

Longitudinal Changes in White Matter Fractional Anisotropy in Adult-Onset Niemann-Pick Disease Type C Patients Treated with Miglustat

**Elizabeth A. Bowman · Dennis Velakoulis ·
Patricia Desmond · Mark Walterfang**

Received: 14 November 2016 / Revised: 18 June 2017 / Accepted: 22 June 2017 / Published online: 15 July 2017
© SSIEM and Springer-Verlag Berlin Heidelberg 2017

Abstract Niemann-Pick disease type C (NPC) is a rare neurometabolic disorder resulting in impaired intracellular lipid trafficking. The only disease-modifying treatment currently available is miglustat, an iminosugar that inhibits the accumulation of lipid metabolites in neurons and other cells. This longitudinal diffusion tensor imaging (DTI) study examined how the rate of white matter change differed between treated and non-treated adult-onset NPC patient groups. Nine adult-onset NPC patients (seven undergoing treatment with miglustat, two not treated) underwent DTI neuroimaging. Rates of change in white matter structure as indexed by Tract-Based Spatial Statistics (TBSS) of fractional anisotropy were compared between treated and untreated patients. Treated patients were found to have a significantly slower rate of white matter change in the corticospinal tracts, the thalamic radiation and the inferior longitudinal fasciculus. This is further evidence that miglustat treatment may have a protective effect on white matter structure in the adult-onset form of the disease.

Communicated by: Marc Patterson

E.A. Bowman
Brain, Mind and Markets Laboratory, University of Melbourne, Melbourne, VIC, Australia

D. Velakoulis · M. Walterfang (✉)
Neuropsychiatry Unit, Royal Melbourne Hospital, Melbourne, VIC, Australia
e-mail: mark.walterfang@gmail.com

D. Velakoulis · M. Walterfang
Melbourne Neuropsychiatry Centre, University of Melbourne, Melbourne, VIC, Australia

P. Desmond
Department of Radiology, University of Melbourne, Melbourne, VIC, Australia

P. Desmond
Department of Radiology, Royal Melbourne Hospital, Melbourne, VIC, Australia

M. Walterfang
Florey Institute of Neurosciences and Mental Health, Melbourne, VIC, Australia

Introduction

Niemann-Pick disease type C (NPC) is a rare, autosomal recessive, neurovisceral disorder involving alterations in intracellular lipid trafficking. Mutations in the NPC1 or the NPC2 genes result in impaired sterol cycling and accumulation of glycosphingolipids and unesterified cholesterol in neural and other tissues. The adult-onset form often presents with psychiatric symptoms, including psychosis, depression and cognitive difficulties (Walterfang et al. 2006). Progressive neurological symptoms include dysphagia, dysarthria and ataxia, and loss of first vertical, then horizontal, saccades (Sevin et al. 2007).

The accumulation of lipids in neurons results in changes to dendritic and axonal morphology (Zervas et al. 2001). Axonal transport mechanisms are also altered, and hyperphosphorylated tau accumulates within neurons (Suzuki et al. 1995). Cerebellar purkinje cells are particularly vulnerable to the damaging effects of accumulated GM2 and GM3 gangliosides. Murine models have found that some cerebellar purkinje populations last longer than others, with those in the cerebellar vermis generally the last to be affected (Taniguchi et al. 2001). Cross-sectional MRI investigations in humans with adult-onset NPC have found significant reductions in thalamic and hippocampal volumes, and both cerebellar grey and white matter volumes compared to age- and gender-matched controls (Walterfang et al. 2010, 2013).

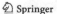

Currently, the only disease-specific treatment for NPC is the iminosugar, miglustat, an inhibitor of glucosylceramide synthase. This reduces glycolipid storage in neurons and has been shown in a controlled clinical trial of juvenile, adolescent and adult-onset NPC to slow disease course (Patterson et al. 2007). Feline models of NPC have found increased purkinje cell survival in the cerebella of treated cats (Stein et al. 2012; Zervas et al. 2001).

Although there have been a number of human neuroimaging studies of NPC, there have been few longitudinal studies. To date, three longitudinal studies have been able to use brain imaging methods, including volumetric methods, diffusion tensor imaging and spectroscopy, to examine treated and untreated patient groups (Bowman et al. 2015; Masingue et al. 2017; Sedel et al. 2016); these have shown a restoration of abnormal markers of neuronal loss and axonal integrity, and a slowing of cerebellar volumetric changes, respectively. A diffusion tensor-based analysis of one patient treated with miglustat suggested a reduction in white matter abnormalities after 1 year of treatment (Scheel et al. 2010), and a French study that examined 11 patients over time showed an improvement in FA in the callosum and corona radiata (Masingue et al. 2017), although no control sample of untreated NPC patients was used.

In the current study, a diffusion-weighted imaging analysis was undertaken using FSL's Tract-Based Spatial Statistics (TBSS) package to explore possible differences in the rate of change in fractional anisotropy (FA) between treated and untreated NPC patients.

Methods

Nine adult-onset NPC patients (five male, four female) were recruited and scanned at the Royal Melbourne Hospital, Melbourne, Australia between 2000 and 2012. The clinical and imaging data are demonstrated in Table 1. The mean age of the patients at baseline was 33.2 years (SD 9.8 years), with mean age of onset of neurological symptoms 27.9 years (SD 10.7 years). NPC diagnosis was confirmed with biochemical analysis of fibroblasts cultured from skin biopsies, including cholesterol esterification rate and staining of perinuclear cholesterol. Further details of patient characteristics can be found in Bowman et al. (2015).

Seven NPC patients received miglustat treatment from baseline. Pre-treatment MRI data points were available for one patient (Patient 3), and one patient refused miglustat treatment and thus served as a natural control (Patient 7). Oral miglustat treatment consisted of 200 mg tds, with the exception of one patient who received 100 mg tds (Patient 9). Three patients (Patients 3, 5 and 6) received oral atypical antipsychotics from baseline and throughout the follow-up period. Patient 3 received 10–30 mg/day and Patient 6 received 30–50 mg/day olanzapine. Patient 5

Table 1 Genetic, clinical and imaging details of treated and untreated patients

Treated patients	Diagnosis	Age at baseline/age at final follow-up (years)	Follow-up period (months)	Scan intervals (months from baseline)	Gender	Age of neurological onset
1	Filipin: variant	49.3/52.2	34	0, 7, 13, 26, 34	M	47.0
2	Genetic: S940L S954L	34.7/36.9	21	0, 6, 13, 21	F	29.0
3	Filipin: variant	34.5/38.3	45	0, 6, 14, 22, 30, 37, 45	F	26.0
4	Genetic: G992R R1186H	45.4/47.8	29	0, 9, 15, 29	F	41.0
5	Genetic: G992R c.3591+4delA	21.1/25.4	52	0, 7, 12, 19, 25, 32, 40, 52	M	19.0
6	Genetic: R518W N1156S	32.8/34.0	14	22, 28, 36	M	25.0
8	Genetic: I1061T I1061T	18.6/23.5	58	0, 10, 15, 18, 22, 26, 31, 38, 46, 58	M	14.0
9	Genetic: R518W N1156S	35.2/36.1	11	0, 11	F	31.0
Untreated patient						
Pre-Tx 6	Genetic: R518W N1156S	31.0/31.5	6	0, 6	M	25.0
7	Genetic: G992R R1186H	31.2/33.1	23	0, 23	M	19.0

received 100 mg/day quetiapine. Additionally, Patient 7 was receiving 500 mg/day oral sodium valproate.

Diffusion tensor imaging (DTI) was undertaken via a 25-direction (one b0 image) echoplanar imaging sequence with 20 axial 5-mm slices, a b-value of 1,000, TE/TR 90/6,000 ms a flip angle of 90°, a matrix size of 256×256 and voxel dimensions of 0.938×0.938 mm.

Participants' fractional anisotropy (FA) maps were aligned into a common space using FSL's FNIRT registration package (Smith et al. 2004). A mean FA image was then created and thinned, to isolate a mean "skeleton" of white matter tracts common to all participants. All skeletonised FA (sFA) images were then aligned to the mean skeleton, creating a skeleton for each participant at each time point. Rate of change of FA over time in each patient was calculated as the beta coefficient of the linear regression of the skeletonised FA data across time. Linear regression across the four-dimensional skeletonised data was performed using the polyfit function in MATLAB. This produced a skeleton for each patient containing the rate of change of white matter FA over time in each voxel. Between-group analysis was performed on these skeletons using Randomise in FSL. Randomise uses permutation-based non-parametric inference using a general linear model design (Winkler et al. 2014). Images were prepared using FSL's Threshold-Free Cluster Enhancement (TFCE) at $p = 0.95$.

Results

A number of regions were identified where in untreated NPC patients' fractional anisotropy was changing significantly faster than in treated patients. These include the corticospinal tracts, the thalamic radiation and the inferior longitudinal fasciculus (Fig. 1).

Discussion

Previous cross-sectional studies have found significant differences in fractional anisotropy between adult-onset NPC patients and age-matched controls (Walterfang et al. 2010; Masingue et al. 2017). Bilateral widespread reductions were found in most major white-matter tracts in the patient groups, including in both projection and association fibres. The thickness and shape of the corpus callosum are also found to be significantly reduced in NPC patients compared to control groups, and the degree of these changes correlated with illness measures in both adult (Walterfang et al. 2011) and paediatric (Lee et al. 2014) patients. One of the few longitudinal studies of NPC disease progression in treated and untreated patients found

that cerebellar white matter was lost at a significantly faster rate in untreated patients than in patients treated with miglustat (Bowman et al. 2015). Similarly, a magnetic resonance spectroscopy (MRS) study in treated and untreated patients found a normalisation of the Cho/NAA ratio in the white matter of the centrum ovale with miglustat treatment (Sedel et al. 2016).

Axonal structure is known to be altered in NPC and can include axonal swelling, spheroid formation and abnormal axonal branching and growth of collaterals (March et al. 1997; Sarna et al. 2003; Zervas et al. 2001). Such disruptions to healthy axonal growth may reflect the abnormal transport of cholesterol and other lipid products to distal axons. Studies have also found a reduction in myelin-specific proteins that may suggest a disruption to myelin-producing biochemical pathways in oligodendrocytes (German et al. 2002; Goodrum and Pentchev 1997).

Miglustat decreases abnormal and destructive glycolipid storage in intracellular compartments through the inhibition of glycosylceramide synthase, and thus the reduction in ultrastructural changes to axons and impairments in myelination may be how treatment with miglustat impacts upon white matter changes in the NPC patient group.

The results of this investigation, the only study to statistically compare both treated and untreated patients over time, reveal that white matter change over time as measured by fractional anisotropy is significantly slower in NPC patients treated with miglustat compared to untreated patients, and is concordant with previous findings suggesting that it slows cerebellar volume loss. Whilst our study is limited by its small sample size, the statistical significance of our results in even this modest sample suggest that this is a true biological effect of treatment, and larger samples may yet demonstrate a more widespread and obvious protective effect on white matter structures from miglustat treatment.

Synopsis

Treatment with miglustat may affect the rate of alteration of white matter structure in progression of Niemann-Pick disease type C.

Author Contributions

Mark Walterfang designed, conceived and implemented the study, including patient recruitment, assessment and data collection. Elizabeth Bowman analysed neuroimaging data. Patricia Desmond assisted with study design and data collection. Dennis Velakoulis assisted with study design and implementation. All authors contributed to preparation and finalisation of the submitted manuscript.

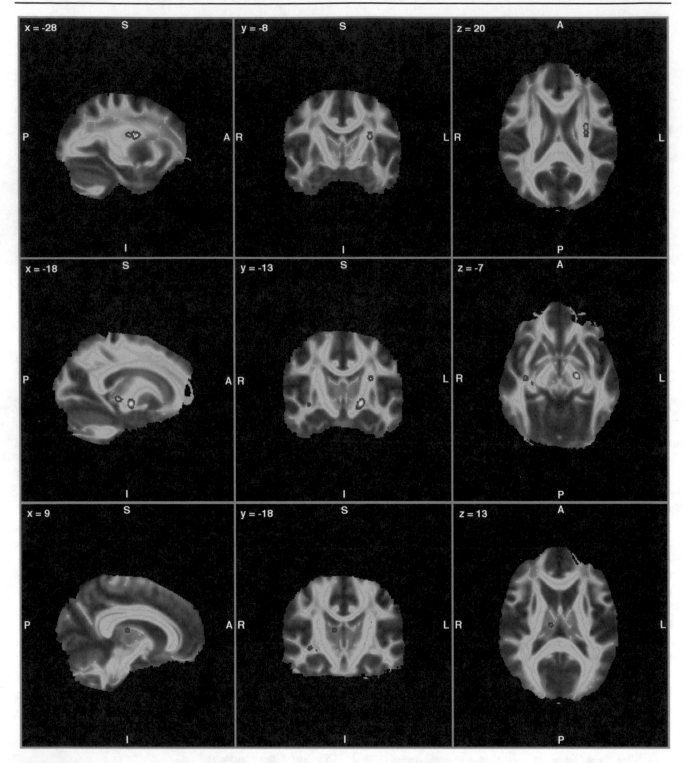

Fig. 1 Areas of difference in treated vs untreated patients. Areas of significantly decreased rate of change in FA in treated compared to untreated patients. The *left column* shows sagittal, *middle column* coronal and *right column* axial images. The *top row* demonstrates a significant difference in the left corticospinal tract, the *middle row* showing changes in the left corticospinal tract and the right inferior longitudinal fasciculus and the *bottom row* demonstrating significantly different change over time in the right thalamic radiation and the right inferior longitudinal fasciculus

Corresponding Author

Mark Walterfang accepts full responsibility for this work, the conduct of the study, had access to the data and controlled the decision to publish.

Competing Interests

Mark Walterfang has served on a scientific advisory board and as a consultant for and received funding for travel from Actelion Pharmaceuticals Ltd, the manufacturer of miglustat. Elizabeth Bowman has received salary support through an unrestricted educational grant to the University of Melbourne from Actelion Pharmaceuticals Ltd. Patricia Desmond and Dennis Velakoulis declare no competing interests.

Funding

This study was supported by an unrestricted educational grant from Actelion Pharmaceuticals. The authors confirm independence from the sponsor; the content of the chapter has not been influenced by this sponsor.

Ethics Approval and Patient Consent

This study was approved by the Melbourne Health Research and Ethics Committee. All subjects provided informed consent.

References

Bowman EA et al (2015) Longitudinal changes in cerebellar and subcortical volumes in adult-onset Niemann-Pick disease type C patients treated with miglustat. J Neurol 262:2106–2114

German DC et al (2002) Neurodegeneration in the Niemann-Pick C mouse: glial involvement. Neuroscience 109:437–450

Goodrum JF, Pentchev PG (1997) Cholesterol reutilization during myelination of regenerating PNS axons is impaired in Niemann-Pick disease type C mice. J Neurosci Res 49:389–392

Lee R et al (2014) Corpus callosum diffusion tensor imaging and volume measures are associated with disease severity in pediatric Niemann-Pick disease type C1. Pediatr Neurol 51:669–674. e5

March PA et al (1997) GABAergic neuroaxonal dystrophy and other cytopathological alterations in feline Niemann-Pick disease type C. Acta Neuropathol 94:164–172

Masingue M et al (2017) Evolution of structural neuroimaging biomarkers in a series of adult patients with Niemann-Pick type C under treatment. Orphanet J Rare Dis 12:22

Patterson MC et al (2007) Miglustat for treatment of Niemann-Pick C disease: a randomised controlled study. Lancet Neurol 6:765–772

Sarna JR et al (2003) Patterned purkinje cell degeneration in mouse models of Niemann-Pick type C disease. J Comp Neurol 456:279–291

Scheel M et al (2010) Eye movement and diffusion tensor imaging analysis of treatment effects in a Niemann-Pick Type C patient. Mol Genet Metab 99(3):291–295

Sedel F et al (2016) Normalisation of brain spectroscopy findings in Niemann-Pick disease type C patients treated with miglustat. J Neurol 263:927–936

Sevin M et al (2007) The adult form of Niemann-Pick disease type C. Brain 130:120–133

Smith SM et al (2004) Advances in functional and structural MR image analysis and implementation as FSL. NeuroImage 23 (Suppl 1):S208–S219

Stein VM et al (2012) Miglustat improves purkinje cell survival and alters microglial phenotype in feline Niemann-Pick disease type C. J Neuropathol Exp Neurol 71:434–448

Suzuki K et al (1995) Neurofibrillary tangles in Niemann-Pick disease type C. Acta Neuropathol 89:227–238

Taniguchi M et al (2001) Sites and temporal changes of gangliosides GM1/GM2 storage in the Niemann-Pick disease type C mouse brain. Brain and Development 23:414–421

Walterfang M et al (2006) The neuropsychiatry of Niemann-Pick type C disease in adulthood. J Neuropsychiatry Clin Neurosci 18:158–170

Walterfang M et al (2010) White and gray matter alterations in adults with Niemann-Pick disease type C: a cross-sectional study. Neurology 75:49–56

Walterfang M et al (2011) Size and shape of the corpus callosum in adult Niemann-Pick type C reflects state and trait illness variables. AJNR Am J Neuroradiol 32:1340–1346

Walterfang M et al (2013) Cerebellar volume correlates with saccadic gain and ataxia in adult Niemann-Pick type C. Mol Genet Metab 108:85–89

Winkler AM et al (2014) Permutation inference for the general linear model. NeuroImage 92:381–397

Zervas M et al (2001) Neurons in Niemann-Pick disease type C accumulate gangliosides as well as unesterified cholesterol and undergo dendritic and axonal alterations. J Neuropathol Exp Neurol 60:49–64

JIMD Reports
DOI 10.1007/8904_2017_45

RESEARCH REPORT

Beta-Ketothiolase Deficiency Presenting with Metabolic Stroke After a Normal Newborn Screen in Two Individuals

Monica H. Wojcik · Klaas J. Wierenga ·
Lance H. Rodan · Inderneel Sahai ·
Sacha Ferdinandusse · Casie A. Genetti ·
Meghan C. Towne · Roy W. A. Peake ·
Philip M. James · Alan H. Beggs ·
Catherine A. Brownstein · Gerard T. Berry ·
Pankaj B. Agrawal

Received: 28 March 2017 / Revised: 16 June 2017 / Accepted: 26 June 2017 / Published online: 20 July 2017
© SSIEM and Springer-Verlag Berlin Heidelberg 2017

Abstract Beta-ketothiolase (mitochondrial acetoacetyl-CoA thiolase) deficiency is a genetic disorder characterized by impaired isoleucine catabolism and ketone body utilization that predisposes to episodic ketoacidosis. It results from biallelic pathogenic variants in the *ACAT1* gene, encoding mitochondrial beta-ketothiolase. We report two cases of beta-ketothiolase deficiency presenting with acute ketoacidosis and "metabolic stroke." The first patient presented at 28 months of age with metabolic acidosis and pallidal stroke in the setting of a febrile gastrointestinal illness. Although 2-methyl-3-hydroxybutyric acid and trace quantities of tiglylglycine were present in urine, a diagnosis of glutaric acidemia type I was initially suspected due to the presence of glutaric and 3-hydroxyglutaric acids. A diagnosis of beta-ketothiolase deficiency was ultimately made through whole exome sequencing which revealed compound heterozygous variants in *ACAT1*. Fibroblast studies for beta-ketothiolase enzyme activity were confirmatory. The second patient presented at 6 months of age with ketoacidosis, and was found to have elevations of urinary 2-methyl-3-hydroxybutyric acid, 2-methylacetoacetic acid, and tiglylglycine. Sequencing of *ACAT1* demonstrated compound heterozygous presumed causative variants. The patient exhibited choreoathethosis 2 months after the acute metabolic decompensation. These cases highlight that, similar to a number of other organic acidemias and mitochondrial disorders, beta-ketothiolase deficiency can present with metabolic stroke. They also illustrate the variability in clinical presentation, imaging, and biochemical evaluation that make screening for and diagnosis of this rare disorder challenging, and further demonstrate the value of whole exome sequencing in the diagnosis of metabolic disorders.

Communicated by: Frits Wijburg

M.H. Wojcik (✉) · P.B. Agrawal (✉)
Division of Newborn Medicine, Boston Children's Hospital and Harvard Medical School, 300 Longwood Avenue, Boston, MA 02115, USA
e-mail: monica.wojcik@childrens.harvard.edu; pagrawal@enders.tch.harvard.edu

M.H. Wojcik · L.H. Rodan · C.A. Genetti · M.C. Towne ·
R.W.A. Peake · P.M. James · A.H. Beggs · C.A. Brownstein ·
G.T. Berry · P.B. Agrawal
Division of Genetics and Genomics, Boston Children's Hospital and Harvard Medical School, Boston, MA, USA

M.H. Wojcik · L.H. Rodan · C.A. Genetti · M.C. Towne · A.H. Beggs ·
C.A. Brownstein · G.T. Berry · P.B. Agrawal
The Manton Center for Orphan Disease Research, Boston Children's Hospital and Harvard Medical School, Boston, MA, USA

K.J. Wierenga
Department of Pediatrics, Section of Genetics, Oklahoma University Health Sciences Center, Oklahoma City, OK, USA

I. Sahai
New England Newborn Screening Program, University of Massachusetts Medical School, Worcester, MA, USA

S. Ferdinandusse
Laboratory Genetic Metabolic Diseases, Department of Clinical Chemistry, Academic Medical Center, Amsterdam, The Netherlands

P.M. James
Division of Genetics and Metabolism, Phoenix Children's Hospital, Phoenix, AZ, USA

Introduction

Beta-ketothiolase deficiency is a rare disorder of ketone body and isoleucine metabolism (Fig. 1). This disorder was first reported in a patient with recurrent metabolic acidosis (Daum et al. 1971). Another early report of a patient with "ketotic hyperglycinemia syndrome" identified a defect in the reaction converting 2-methylacetoacetyl-CoA to propionyl-CoA and acetyl-CoA with increased amounts of 2-methyl-3-hydroxybutyric acid, 2-methylacetoacetic acid, and butanone excreted in urine (Hillman and Keating 1974). Beta-ketothiolase has since been identified as the only enzyme able to convert 2-methylacetoacetyl-CoA to propionyl-CoA and acetyl-CoA (Middleton and Bartlett 1983). The beta-ketothiolase enzyme is encoded by *ACAT1*, and the disorder follows autosomal recessive inheritance.

Patients with beta-ketothiolase deficiency typically present in early childhood with acute and recurrent ketoacidosis following an illness (Korman 2006). They are typically asymptomatic between episodes of metabolic decompensation (Fukao et al. 2014), which generally decrease in frequency with age. Similar to a number of other organic acidemias and mitochondrial disorders, beta-ketothiolase deficiency can present with metabolic stroke and associated neurological sequelae (Ozand et al. 1994; Buhas et al. 2013; O'Neill et al. 2014; Yalcinkaya et al. 2001; Shiasi Arani and Soltani 2014; Akella et al. 2014). Acute treatment of ketoacidosis in this disorder typically consists of a high dextrose intravenous (IV) infusion, correction of the metabolic acidosis with bicarbonate, and carnitine supplementation if deficient. Chronic management involves avoiding prolonged periods of fasting and potential dietary modifications including mild protein restriction and carnitine supplementation, if deficient.

We present two patients with beta-ketothiolase deficiency both presenting with ketoacidosis and acute neurological events. Neither case was detected on routine newborn screening. These cases highlight variability in the clinical presentation, imaging, and biochemical evaluation that make screening for and diagnosis of this disorder challenging.

Materials and Methods

Patient One

A 28-month-old girl presented with a decreased level of consciousness, hypoglycemia, and profound metabolic acidosis in the setting of an infectious gastrointestinal illness with 2 days of emesis and decreased oral intake. On the day of admission, she was found unresponsive by her parents. Initial blood glucose was 42 mg/dL (reference interval: 40–100). Venous blood gas was notable for pH of 6.87 (reference interval: 7.35–7.45), pCO_2 of 23 mmHg (reference interval: 35–45), and measured bicarbonate of less than 5 mmol/L (reference interval: 20–33). Urine ketones were estimated to be greater than 80 mg/dL by dipstick. She was intubated and administered IV boluses of dextrose, normal saline, and sodium bicarbonate and was admitted to the intensive care unit. Brain magnetic resonance imaging (MRI) showed bilateral T2 hyperinten-

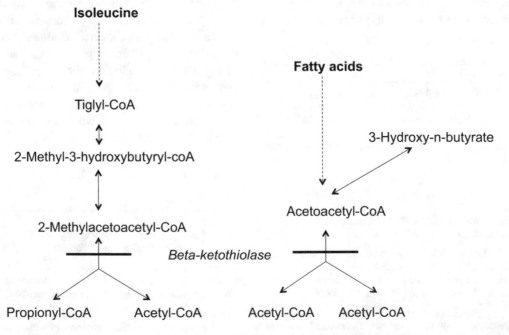

Fig. 1 Beta-ketothiolase deficiency. The location of the metabolic defect is indicated by the solid bar

sity and reduced diffusivity in the globus pallidi and substantia nigra (Fig. 2).

Prior to this admission, the child had been healthy and developing normally. She had a history of preterm birth at

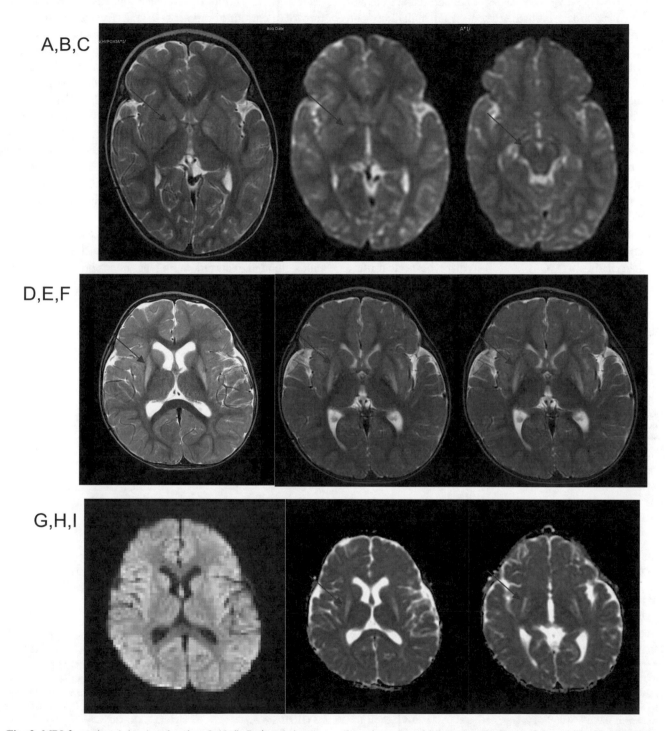

Fig. 2 MRI for patient 1 (**a–c**) and patient 2 (**d–i**). Patient 1, images obtained at 2 years of age: (**a**) Axial T2-weighted MR demonstrates T2 hyperintensity of bilateral globus pallidi. (**b, c**) Diffusion-weighted imaging (DWI) demonstrates bilaterally restricted diffusion in globus pallidi and substantia nigra (*arrows*). Patient 2, images obtained at 14 months of age: (**d–f**) Axial T2-weighted MRI demonstrates T2 hyperintensity of bilateral putamina, and to a lesser degree globus pallidi (*arrows*). (**g**) Diffusion-weighted imaging (DWI) and (**h, i**) apparent diffusion coefficient (ADC) sequences demonstrate that regions of signal change in putamina and globus pallidi lack restricted diffusion

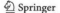

32 weeks gestational age. Two newborn screening (NBS) specimens had been collected from the infant on day of life (DOL) 3 and 13 and both were reported as normal (Table 1).

The metabolism service was consulted and recommended IV 10% dextrose with half-normal sodium acetate and sodium bicarbonate boluses. Based on an initial suspicon for an organic acidemia, she was empirically treated with intramuscular cyanocobalamin and enteral levocarnitine and riboflavin.

Initial qualitative assessment of urine organic acids was notable for marked ketosis, with large peaks of 3-hydroxybutyric and acetoacetic acids predominating. There was also a medium-chain dicarboxylic aciduria, with significant quantities of adipic acid together with smaller amounts of suberic, sebacic, and 3-hydroxysebacic acids in a pattern consistent with physiologic ketosis. Also notable were the presence of significant quantities of 2-methyl-3-hydroxbutyric and glutaric acids, together with trace quantities of both tiglylglycine and 3-hydroxyglutaric acid. Plasma acylcarnitine analysis demonstrated increases in acetylcarnitine (C2) and 3-hydroxybutyrylcarnitine

(C4OH), a pattern consistent with physiologic ketosis. Notably, concentrations of 2-methyl-3-hydroxybutyrylcarnitine (C5OH) and tiglylcarnitine (C5:1) were within the reference intervals. Plasma free carnitine was mildly decreased (22.4 μmol/L; reference interval: 26–60) with a free/total carnitine ratio of 0.31% (reference interval: 0.50–0.90). Plasma amino acid analysis produced a pattern suggestive of an acute catabolic state, with moderate increases in the branched chain amino acids. A plasma glutaric acid level, collected on the day of admission, was elevated at 1,088 ng/mL (reference interval: <250). Plasma 3-hydroxyglutaric acid was also elevated at 198 ng/mL (reference interval: <65). Cerebrospinal fluid (CSF) glutaric acid was normal at 98 ng/mL (reference interval: <250) with increased CSF 3-hydroxyglutaric acid at 121 ng/mL (reference interval: <65). Based on these results, a presumptive diagnosis of glutaric acidemia type I (GA I) was made.

The patient's metabolic acidosis and ketosis improved over the first hospital day on high-dextrose containing fluids, though recurred during an interruption in her IV

Table 1 Concentration of acylcarnitines and ratios relevant for profiling beta-ketothiolase in the newborn screening specimens from patient 1

Relevant acylcarnitines/ ratios	Specimen 1–DOL 3 Original Value	Original Z-score	Retest Value	Retest Z-score	Specimen 2–DOL 13 Original Value	Original Z-score	Retest Value	Retest Z-score	MA cut-off	CLR tools 99th %ile of normal	1st %ile of BKT	5th %ile of BKT	Target cut-offs
C5:1	0.04	3.34	0.05	3.98	0.05	3.98	0.04	3.34	0.08	0.06	0.07	0.15	0.06–0.15
C5OH	0.18	1.44	0.16	1.09	0.14	0.7	0.18	1.44	0.8	0.36	0.49	0.65	0.36–0.82
C4OH	–	–	0.1	–0.48	–	–	0.1	–0.48	0.75	0.47	0.58	0.6	0.47–0.81
C0	29.41	0.74	55.52	2.59	26.01	0.38	28.27	0.63	–	50.55	9.3	11.19	–
C5	0.37	2.5	0.27	1.52	0.33	2.14	0.38	2.58	–	0.38	0.1	0.13	–
C8	0.06	–1.21	0.05	–1.86	0.1	0.61	0.09	0.24	–	0.17	0.03	0.04	–
C16	1.88	–1.44	1.72	–1.7	0.74	–4.18	0.63	–4.65	–	5.73	1.13	1.32	–
C5OH × C5:1	0.007	3.08	0.008	3.28	0.007	3.08	0.007	3.08	0.02	–	–	–	–
C5 × C5:1/ C5OH	0.082	2.83	0.084	2.88	0.118	3.52	0.084	2.88	0.05	–	–	–	–
C5OH/C8	2.74	1.77	3.16	2.12	1.40	0.22	2.00	1.01	10	7.81	3.68	4.95	7.81–10
C5OH/C0	0.006	–	0.002	–	0.005	–	0.006	–	–	0.02	0.02	0.02	0.018–0.026
C4OH/C16	–	–	0.06	–	–	–	0.16	–	–	0.13	0.27	0.28	0.13–0.28

BKT beta-ketothiolase deficiency. Concentrations and values shown are those reported originally and after retesting after diagnosis (at time of retest additional markers including C4OH were also being analyzed for routine screening). Values for the 99th percentile of the normal population, and the 1st & 5th percentiles in confirmed BKT cases, and recommended cut-offs for the relevant markers and ratios in the CLIR-R4S database are shown [http://www.clir-r4s.org/; accessed 05/22/2017]. C5:1, C5OH and C4OH are expected to be high in BKT. C0, C5, C8, and C16 are utilized for calculating ratios and scores to risks of BKT by the NBS Analytical Tools in the CLIR-R4S databases and by the New England Newborn Screening Program (NENSP). C5OH × C5:1, [C5 × C5:1/C5OH] and C5OH/C8 are utilized by NENSP for evaluating BKT profiles/ risk of disorder. C5OH/C8, C5OH/C0 and C4OH/C16 are required by calculating a score/risk of disorder by the CLIR-R4S in the current BKT Post-Analytic Tool [BKT 009 2012-01-08 Single-D]. The score for patient 1 calculated using the BKT Post-Analytic Tool was "0" in both specimens with the interpretation "Score Profile is not informative for BKT"

fluids and enteral nutrition. Repeat plasma and urine glutaric acid and 3-hydroxyglutaric acid levels obtained during the hospitalization were normal.

Clinically, her level of consciousness improved and she was extubated on hospital day four. She was noted to have generalized athetosis and dystonia, particularly affecting her left leg. She was started on baclofen, trihexyphenidyl, gabapentin, melatonin, and clonazepam. Due to the suspicion for (GA I), a diet low in tryptophan and lysine was initiated.

Enzyme analysis of glutaryl-CoA dehydrogenase was performed in cultured skin fibroblasts and was normal. Sequencing of *GCDH* for GA I was negative. Additionally, mitochondrial genome screening and sequencing of *SURF1*, *SCO2*, and *COX10* to evaluate for mitochondrial disorders were unremarkable. She was transitioned back to a regular diet and riboflavin and levocarnitine supplements were discontinued. A follow-up urine collected approximately 1 week later was essentially normal, with only trace levels of 2-methyl-3-hydroxybutyric and 3-hydroxybutyric acids and the medium-chain dicarboxylic acids noted. During subsequent hospital presentations for fever and emesis, she was found to have normal or mildly elevated plasma and urine glutaric and 3-hydroxyglutaric acids, and qualitative urine organic acid profiles that were either normal or consistent with ketosis with trace levels of 2-methyl-3-hydroxybutyric acid.

Her dystonia gradually improved and she was ultimately weaned off baclofen, gabapentin, trihexyphenidyl, clonazepam, and melatonin. At present, she is developmentally normal with spasticity of the lower extremities and occasional dyskinesia of the upper extremities.

Patient 2

A 6-month-old male infant was seen by his pediatrician in the setting of 2 days of nasal congestion and otitis media. The following day, he presented to the emergency department with lethargy and Kussmaul respirations and was found to have severe ketoacidosis, with a blood gas notable for a pH of 7.07, calculated bicarbonate of 3 mmol/L, and base excess −27. Urinalysis showed 4+ ketones by dipstick. He was given an IV fluid bolus and admitted to the intensive care unit.

Prior to this presentation, the patient had been developing normally. At 3 months of age, he had a focal seizure of unclear etiology. Electroencephalogram, head CT, and brain MRI prior to his metabolic decompensation were normal.

Infectious studies returned positive for adenovirus. Urine organic acids showed marked excretion of 3-hydroxybuty-ric acid, acetoacetic acid, lactic acid, 2-methyl-3-hydroxybutyric acid and 2-methylacetoacetic acid, and trace excretion of tiglylglycine. A plasma acylcarnitine profile revealed elevated C2 and markedly elevated C4OH with normal C5OH and C5:1. Plasma-free carnitine was decreased at 15 μmol/L and total carnitine was normal. Plasma amino acids and urine acylglycines were unremarkable.

He was administered IV levocarnitine while inpatient, and switched to oral levocarnitine for home. He also received high-dextrose IV fluids containing sodium bicarbonate. His severe ketoacidosis persisted for 24 h and then slowly improved, normalizing on the third hospital day.

At a follow-up visit 2 months after his hospitalization, it was noted that the patient had not attained any further developmental milestones. Three months after his hospitalization, at 8 months of age, he was found to have near continuous choreoathetoid movements of his extremities. Brain MRI at 14 months of age demonstrated interval development of increased T2 signal of the bilateral lentiform nuclei, as well as scattered foci of increased T2 signal in the periventricular and subcortical white matter (Fig. 2).

The patient has not since presented with any episodes of ketoacidosis. He continues to receive physical, occupational, and speech therapy and his oral intake remains poor. Clonazepam was tried, but appeared to decrease his appetite even more and did not improve his movement disorder.

Whole Exome Sequencing (Patient 1)

Total genomic DNA was extracted from peripheral blood mononuclear cells using QIAmp DNA Mini Kit (Qiagen). DNA from the proband and both biological parents was sent for whole exome sequencing (WES). WES was provided by the Yale University Center for Mendelian Genomics on an Illumina HiSeq 2000 instrument with blood samples pooled 6 per lane. Libraries (TruSeq DNA v2 Sample Preparation kit; Illumina, San Diego, CA) and whole exome capture (EZ Exome 2.0, Roche) were performed according to manufacturer protocols. FASTQs were filtered, aligned, and variants were filtered and annotated by Codified Genomics (proprietary algorithm, Houston, TX). Sanger confirmation of the candidate variant was performed at the Boston Children's Hospital Manton Center Gene Discovery Core. Likely pathogenic variants were selected to include nonsynonymous, splice site, and indel variants with an allele frequency <1% in the NHLBI exome variant server database (http://evs.gs.washington.edu/EVS/) or 1000 genomes project (http://www.1000genomes.org) and were evaluated in the ExAC database (http://www.exac.broadinstitute.org). The pathogenicity of the variants was evaluated in silico using Polyphen-2, SIFT, and MutationTaster.

ACAT1 Gene Sequencing (Patient 2)

ACAT1 was clinically sequenced using standard PCR and sequencing methods.

Beta-Ketothiolase Enzyme Activity Measurement (Patient 1)

Beta-ketothiolase enzyme activity was measured in a fibroblast homogenate prepared in phosphate buffered saline by sonication. 2-Methylacetoacetyl-CoA was used as substrate in the reaction in the presence of CoA. After termination of the reaction, substrate and product (propionyl-CoA) were separated by ultra-high pressure liquid chromatography.

Results

Patient 1

WES revealed 470 variants that satisfied the frequency filtration criteria. Of these, 26 were either de novo dominant or recessive (homozygous or compound heterozygous in trans). Genes overlapping those variants were further evaluated for human disease or animal models consistent with the phenotype and only one gene, *ACAT1*, fulfilled the criteria. A splicing variant, c.1006-1G>C, was maternally inherited while a missense variant, c.1160T>C, p.Ile387Thr, was paternally inherited. The splicing variant has been previously reported as pathogenic (Fukao et al. 1992a) and is not seen in ExAC database (Lek 2016). The missense variant c.1160T>C occurs at a highly conserved position, is seen in only four individuals in ExAC, all heterozygous (mean allele frequency or MAF <0.003%), and is predicted to be pathogenic by several in silico methods including Polyphen-2, SIFT, and MutationTaster.

Analysis of beta-ketothiolase activity in cultured skin fibroblasts from patient 1 confirmed the diagnosis, as the enzyme activity was markedly reduced to below the limit of quantitation of the assay at <1 nmol/(min.mg of protein) [reference interval: 23–74 nmol/(min.mg of protein)].

Patient 2

ACAT1 sequencing revealed bi-allelic mutations, one of which, c.1006-2A>C, has been previously reported as pathogenic (Fukao et al. 1992b) and is seen in only four individuals in ExAC, all heterozygous (MAF <0.003%).

The other, c.299G>A, p.Gly100Glu, is not previously reported but occurs at a highly conserved position, is predicted to be pathogenic by SIFT, Polyphen-2 and MutationTaster, and is not seen in ExAC.

Discussion

Beta-ketothiolase deficiency is an autosomal recessive disorder impairing isoleucine catabolism and ketone body utilization that predisposes to episodic ketoacidosis (Fig. 1). We present two patients with beta-ketothiolase deficiency manifesting with ketoacidosis and neurological injury. The diagnosis in the first patient was not suspected clinically, and in fact biochemical evaluation misdirected the work-up towards GA I, despite the presence of 2-methyl-3-hydroxybutyric acid and trace quantities of tiglylglycine on initial qualitative urine organic acid analysis (although these metabolites were absent from subsequent urine organic acid analyses). "Hypothesis-free" testing with WES was required to make the diagnosis, confirmed by enzyme analysis. The second case showed the classic metabolic profile of beta-ketothiolase deficiency, directing clinicians to the appropriate diagnosis. The dichotomy of these cases serves to highlight the challenges in the biochemical diagnosis of beta-ketothiolase deficiency. The classic metabolic perturbations seen in this disorder, namely elevations of 2-methyl-3-hydroxybutyric acid, 2-methylacetoacetic acid, and tiglylglycine in urine, with C5OH and C5:1 in plasma, may not all be present. This is even more problematic in patients with residual enzyme activity, and during periods of clinical stability (Fukao et al. 2003, 2012; Sarafoglou et al. 2011). In particular, 2-methylacetoacetic acid is unstable and can be difficult to detect with routinely used methods for organic acid analysis (Korman 2006; Catanzano et al. 2010).

Patient 1 was initially suspected to have GA I based on elevations of glutaric acid and 3-hydroxyglutaric acid in urine and 3-hydroxyglutaric acid in CSF during her initial presentation. Both enzymatic and genetic testing for this disorder were entirely normal, arguing against even a carrier state. The explanation for these transient elevations is not clear, but could relate to a generalized mitochondrial dysfunction in the context of her severe metabolic decompensation. It is also worth noting that metabolic stroke in GA I typically involves the striatum, which was entirely spared in our first patient.

Neither case was detected through NBS, which has been previously observed in this disorder (Sarafoglou et al. 2011; Estrella et al. 2014). Rather, both patients were diagnosed after an acute decompensation had already occurred, highlighting the need for improved early diagnosis. Beta-ketothiolase deficiency is diagnosed in many NBS programs through demonstration of increased C5OH and C5:1 levels on a dried blood spot specimen. However, the concentrations of these markers may be normal in affected patients. While the incidence of this disorder has been reported at approximately 1 in 1,000,000, this is widely considered to be an underestimate, and significantly more cases are likely to be detected through expanded NBS programs in the United States. Data from two NBS programs suggest an incidence closer to 1 in 200,000–300,000 (Sarafoglou et al. 2011; Frazier et al. 2006; Abdelkreem et al. 2016). The NBS results for patient 1 were scrutinized closely when she presented clinically, and it was noted that the concentration of C5:1 in the two specimens was in the high normal range in both at 0.04 and 0.05 (reference range <0.08), which at the time was attributed to her prematurity. The concentration of C5OH was normal. C4OH, now routinely analyzed and utilized to evaluate the metabolic profile for beta-ketothiolase deficiency, was not part of the analyses when this infant was originally screened. The original screening specimens were retrieved after the diagnosis of beta-ketothiolase deficiency was confirmed and reanalyzed to evaluate these additional markers (Table 1). Although C5:1 was in high range of normal, the metabolic profile was not suggestive of beta-ketothiolase deficiency. The results were also compared and scored using the Post Analytic Interpretative Tools of the CLIR-R4S collaborative database (Marquardt et al. 2012). The score for patient 1 was "0" in both specimens with the interpretation "Score Profile is not informative for BKT." Notably, the C5:1 concentration in both specimens was below the 1st percentile of C5:1 concentration in confirmed beta-ketothiolase deficiency cases in the database.

Both of the patients that we present developed metabolic stroke, one affecting the globus pallidi and the other the striatum. This variability in the location of metabolic stroke associated with beta-ketothiolase deficiency is consistent with what has been previously described in the literature (Table 2) and is unique amongst organic acidemias since metabolic stroke in these disorders typically shows a striking selective vulnerability for specific structures. Interestingly, patients with 2-methyl-3-hydroxybutyrate dehydrogenase deficiency (HSD10 disease), another disorder of isoleucine metabolism in which elevated 2-methyl 3-hydroxybutyric acid and tiglylglycine are observed, but not 2-methylacetoacetic acid, can present with metabolic stroke affecting the basal ganglia in addition to other abnormalities seen on neuroimaging such as cortical atrophy (Cazorla et al. 2007; Zschocke 2012). The explanation for this variability in metabolic stroke pattern could potentially relate to factors such as central nervous system maturity, modifier genes, or relative accumulation of toxic metabolites. This certainly poses a barrier to MRI pattern recognition of metabolic stroke in this disorder.

In conclusion, we present two individuals with beta-ketothiolase deficiency, illustrating the wide variability in clinical presentation, imaging, and biochemical studies that make diagnosis challenging. The first patient also highlights the utility of WES in the diagnosis of rare inborn errors of metabolism, particularly when biochemical evaluation is non-contributory or incongruent with the clinical picture. A high index of clinical suspicion in the infant or young child presenting with severe ketoacidosis is required for prompt diagnosis and potentially life-saving medical management.

Synopsis

Beta-ketothiolase deficiency, causing episodic, severe ketoacidosis, can present with metabolic stroke and may be difficult to diagnose biochemically.

Monica H. Wojcik conceptualized this case report, contributed to the writing of the manuscript, and provided clinical care for one of the patients reported.

Klaas J. Wierenga provided clinical care for one of the patients reported and contributed to the writing of the manuscript.

Lance H. Rodan provided clinical care for one of the patients reported and contributed to the writing of the manuscript.

Inderneel Sahai performed the newborn screen analysis for one of the patients reported and critically reviewed the manuscript.

Sacha Ferdinandusse performed the fibroblast enzyme assay for one of the patients reported and critically reviewed the manuscript.

Casie A. Genetti contributed to the whole exome sequencing for one of the patients reported.

Meghan C. Towne contributed to the whole exome sequencing for one of the patients reported.

Roy W.A. Peake aided in the biochemical laboratory interpretation for one of the patients reported and critically reviewed the manuscript.

Philip James provided clinical care for one of the patients reported and critically reviewed the manuscript.

Alan H. Beggs contributed to the whole exome sequencing for one of the patients reported and critically reviewed the manuscript.

Catherine A. Brownstein contributed to the whole exome sequencing for one of the patients reported.

Table 2 Brain imaging findings in beta-ketothiolase deficiency

Author	Clinical description	Biochemical abnormalities	Enzyme assay	Molecular genetic diagnosis	Neurologic abnormalities	MRI/CT findings
O'Neill et al. (2014)	5-year-old female presenting with a neurologic decompensation and metabolic acidosis	2-Methylacetoacetate, 2-methyl-3-hydroxybutyrate, tiglylglycine, abnormal acylcarnitine and tiglylcarnitine in urine	Not performed	Homozygous p.I323V	Abnormal posturing	MRI: initially with T2/FLAIR hyperintensities in bilateral globi pallidi with restricted diffusion, repeated 1 year later with no restricted diffusion seen
Buhas et al. (2013)	17-year-old male presenting with hypotonia and abnormal movements	Elevated 2-methyl-3-hydroxybutyrate and 2-methylacetoacetate in urine and elevated plasma C5:1 acylcarnitine	Reduced activity	p.G125A and p.N158D	Developmental delay and neurologic symptoms	MRI: initially with T2 hyperintensities in the bilateral putamen and cerebral peduncles, repeated several years later with atrophy of putamen and T2 hyperintensity of the posterolateral putamen and hyperintensity of the putamen and caudate nuclei on diffusion-weighted imaging
Ozand et al. (1994)	Patient 1: 7-month-old female presenting with ketoacidosis	2-Methyl-acetoacetate, 2-methyl-3-hydroxybutyrate, and tiglylglycine in urine	Absent activity	Not available	Developmental delay	MRI: T2 hyperintensity in bilateral posterolateral putamen into the lower part of the corona radiata
	Patient 2: 7-year-old female evaluated due to diagnosis of BKT deficiency in sibling (patient 1)	2-Methyl-acetoacetate, 2-methyl-3-hydroxybutyrate, and tiglylglycine in urine	Absent activity	Not available	Developmental delay, history of febrile seizure	MRI: lesions in bilateral lentiform nuclei, similar to patient 1
	Patient 3: 8-month-old male presenting with ketoacidosis	2-Methyl-acetoacetate, 2-methyl-3-hydroxybutyrate, and tiglylglycine in urine	Absent activity	Not available	Developmental delay, febrile seizures, and hypotonia	MRI: lesions in external capsule, similar to patient 1
Shiasi Arani and Soltani (2014)	6-month-old male with ketoacidosis	2-Methyl-3-hydroxybutyrate, and tiglylglycine in urine	Not available	Not available	Developmental regression, abnormal tongue movements, dystonia	MRI: hypomyelination of white matter
Akella et al. (2014)	11-month-old male presenting with ketoacidosis	Elevated C5OH and C5:1 on acylcarnitine profile, elevated 2-methyl-3-hydroxybutyrate, 2-methylacetoacetate, and tiglylglycine in urine	Absent activity	Homozygous p.M193R	Developmental regression, dystonia, seizures	CT: hypodensities in bilateral lentiform nuclei and caudate head, later repeated with basal ganglia calcification seen
Yalcinkaya et al. (2001)	7-year-old male presenting with ketoacidosis	2-Methyl-3-hydroxybutyrate and tiglylglycine in urine	Decreased activity	Not available	Dystonia	CT: hypodensities in bilateral globi pallidi; MRI: T2 hyperintensity and T1 hypointensity in bilateral globi pallidi

Gerard T. Berry provided clinical care for one of the patients reported and critically reviewed the manuscript.

Pankaj B. Agrawal conceptualized this case report, contributed to the whole exome sequencing for one of the patients reported, and contributed to the writing of the manuscript.

Corresponding Author

Pankaj B. Agrawal, who serves as guarantor for the chapter, accepts full responsibility for the work, had access to the data, and controlled the decision to publish.

Competing Interests

No competing interests are reported by the authors.

Funding

MHW is supported by training grant T32 HD07466 through the National Institutes of Health (NIH). PBA was supported by R01 AR068429 from the National Institute of Arthritis and Musculoskeletal and Skin Diseases of the NIH and U19 HD077671 from the National Institute of Child Health and Human Development/National Human Genome Research Institute/NIH. The Gene Discovery Core of The Manton Center for Orphan Disease Research, Boston Children's Hospital also supported the work. Whole exome sequencing was performed by the Yale Center for Mendelian Genomics, supported by NIH grant 2UM1HG006504. Sanger sequencing was performed by the Molecular Genetics Core Facility of the Intellectual and Developmental Disabilities Research Center (IDDRC) at Boston Children's Hospital, supported by NIH grant U54 HD090255.

Ethics Approval

As these are retrospective case reports, approval by an Institutional Review Board was not required. Patient one and the patient's parents had whole exome sequencing performed on a research basis through an IRB-approved protocol with the Manton Center for Orphan Disease Research at Boston Children's Hospital.

Patient Consent Statement

As these are retrospective case reports without identifiable information, patient consent was not obtained.

References

Abdelkreem E, Otsuka H, Sasai H et al (2016) Beta-ketothiolase deficiency: resolving challenges in diagnosis. J Inborn Errors Metab Screen 4:1–9

Akella RRD, Aoyama C, Mori C, Lingappa L, Cariappa R, Fukao T (2014) Metabolic encephalopathy in beta-ketothiolase deficiency: the first report from India. Brain Dev 36:537–540

Buhas D, Bernard G, Fukao T, Decarie JC, Chouinard S, Mitchell GA (2013) A treatable new cause of chorea: beta-ketothiolase deficiency. Mov Disord 28:1054–1056

Catanzano F, Ombrone D, Di Stefano C et al (2010) The first case of mitochondrial acetoacetyl-CoA thiolase deficiency identified by expanded newborn metabolic screening in Italy: the importance of an integrated diagnostic approach. J Inherit Metab Dis 33:91

Cazorla MR, Verdu A, Perez-Cerda C, Ribes A (2007) Neuroimage findings in 2-methyl-3-hydroxybutytyl-CoA dehydrogenase deficiency. Pediatr Neurol 36:264–267

Daum RS, Lamm PH, Mamer OA, Scriver CR (1971) A "new" disorder of isoleucine catabolism. Lancet 2:1289–1290

Estrella J, Wilcken B, Carpenter K, Bhattacharya K, Tchan M, Wiley V (2014) Expanded newborn screening in New South Wales: missed cases. J Inherit Metab Dis 37:881–887

Frazier DM, Millington DS, McCandless SE et al (2006) The tandem mass spectrometry newborn screening experience in North Carolina: 1997-2005. J Inherit Metab Dis 29:76–85

Fukao T, Yamaguchi S, Orii T, Osumi T, Hashimoto T (1992a) Molecular basis of 3-ketothiolase deficiency: identification of an AG to AC substitution at the splice acceptor site of intron 10 causing exon 11 skipping. Biochim Biophys Acta 1139:184–188

Fukao T, Yamaguchi S, Orii T, Schutgens RB, Osumi T, Hashimoto T (1992b) Identification of three mutant alleles of the gene for mitochondrial acetoacetyl-coenzyme A thiolase. A complete analysis of two generations of a family with 3-ketothiolase deficiency. J Clin Invest 89:474–479

Fukao T, Zhang GX, Sakura N et al (2003) The mitochondrial acetoacetyl-CoA thiolase (T2) deficiency in Japanese patients: urinary organic acid and blood acylcarnitine profiles under stable conditions have subtle abnormalities in T2-deficient patients with some residual T2 activity. J Inherit Metab Dis 26:423–431

Fukao T, Maruyama S, Ohura T et al (2012) Three Japanese patients with beta-ketothiolase deficiency who share a mutation, C.431A>C (H144P) in ACAT1: subtle abnormality in urinary organic acid analysis and blood acylcarnitine analysis using tandem mass spectrometry. JIMD Reports 3:107–115

Fukao T, Mitchell G, Sass JO, Hori T, Orii K, Aoyama Y (2014) Ketone body metabolism and its defects. J Inherit Metab Dis 37:541–551

Hillman RE, Keating JP (1974) Beta-ketothiolase deficiency as a cause of the "ketotic hyperglycinemia syndrome". Pediatrics 53:221–225

Korman SH (2006) Inborn errors of isoleucine degradation: a review. Mol Genet Metab 89:289–299

Lek M (2016) Analysis of protein-coding genetic variation in 60,706 humans. Nature 536:285–291

Marquardt G, Currier R, McHugh DM et al (2012) Enhanced interpretation of newborn screening results without analyte cutoff values. Genet Med 14:648–655

Middleton B, Bartlett K (1983) The synthesis and characterisation of 2-methylacetoacetyl coenzyme A and its use in the identification of the site of the defect in 2-methylacetoacetic and 2-methyl-3-hydroxybutyric aciduria. Clin Chim Acta 128:291–305

O'Neill ML, Kuo F, Saigal G (2014) MRI of pallidal involvement in beta-ketothiolase deficiency. J Neuroimaging 24:414–417

Ozand PT, Rashed M, Gascon GG et al (1994) 3-Ketothiolase deficiency: a review and four new patients with neurologic symptoms. Brain Dev 16:38–45

Sarafoglou K, Matern D, Redlinger-Grosse K et al (2011) Siblings with mitochondrial acetoacetyl-CoA thiolase deficiency not identified by newborn screening. Pediatrics 128:e246–e250

Shiasi Arani K, Soltani B (2014) First report of 3-oxothiolase deficiency in Iran. Int J Endocrinol Metab 12:e10960

Yalcinkaya C, Apaydin H, Ozekmekci S, Gibson KM (2001) Delayed-onset dystonia associated with 3-oxothiolase deficiency. Mov Disord 16:372–375

Zschocke J (2012) HSD10 disease: clinical consequences of mutations in the HSD17B10 gene. J Inherit Metab Dis 25:81–89

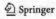

JIMD Reports
DOI 10.1007/8904_2017_46

RESEARCH REPORT

Rapidly Progressive White Matter Involvement in Early Childhood: The Expanding Phenotype of Infantile Onset Pompe?

A. Broomfield · J. Fletcher · P. Hensman · R. Wright ·
H. Prunty · J. Pavaine · S.A. Jones

Received: 2 April 2017 / Revised: 31 May 2017 / Accepted: 30 June 2017 / Published online: 20 July 2017
© SSIEM and Springer-Verlag Berlin Heidelberg 2017

Abstract Glycogen accumulation in the central nervous system of patients with classical infantile onset Pompe disease (IOPD) has been a consistent finding on the few post-mortems performed. While delays in myelination and a possible reduction in processing speed have previously been noted, it has only been recently that the potential for clinically significant progressive white matter disease has been noted. The limited reports thus far published infer that in some IOPD patients, this manifests as intellectual decline in the second decade of life. We present a CRIM negative patient, immunomodulated with rituximab and methotrexate at birth, who despite an initial good clinical response to ERT, at the age of just under 4 years, presented with evolving spasticity in the lower limbs. The investigation of which revealed progressive central nervous system involvement. Given both the earlier onset of the symptoms and consanguineous familial pedigree, extensive biochemical and genetic investigation was undertaken to ensure no alternative pathology was elucidated. In light of these findings, we review the radiology and post-mortems of previous cases and discuss the potential mechanisms that may underlie this presentation.

Introduction

Prior to the advent of enzyme replacement therapy (ERT), patients with the classical infantile onset variant of Pompe disease (IOPD), a lysosomal storage disease due to a deficiency in the enzyme acid α-glucosidase (GAA) (Hers 1963) (OMIM #232300), typically died within the first year of life (van den Hout et al. 2003). The inherent mortality has been predominately attributable to cardiorespiratory failure (Byrne et al. 2011) with both the cardiac hypertrophy and the peripheral myopathy inherent to the excessive skeletal muscle lysosomal glycogen accumulation, being the major causes of morbidity and mortality (Lim et al. 2014).

While glycogen has been demonstrated to accumulate in central neuronal tissue (Gambetti et al. 1971), even prenatally (Chen et al. 2004), its effects have thus far been apparently limited. For although an initial case series of five patients of treated with ERT suggested patients may suffer from delay in CNS myelination, or in one severe case a possible dysmyelination (Chien et al. 2006) the clinical significance of these findings has been unclear, with cognitive outcome over the first decade not overtly

Communicated by: Martina Huemer, MD

A. Broomfield (✉) · J. Fletcher · S.A. Jones
Willink Biochemical Genetics Unit, Manchester Centre for Genomic Medicine, St Mary's Hospital, Central Manchester Foundation Trust, Manchester M13 9WL, UK
e-mail: alexander.broomfield@cmft.nhs.uk

P. Hensman
Department of Physiotherapy, Royal Manchester Children's Hospital, Central Manchester Foundation Trust, Manchester M13 9WL, UK

R. Wright
Manchester Centre for Genomic Medicine, St Mary's Hospital, Central Manchester Foundation Trust, Manchester M13 9WL, UK

H. Prunty
Department of Biochemistry, Great Ormond Street Hospital, Great Ormond Street, London WC1N 3JH, UK

J. Pavaine
Department of Paediatric Neuroradiology, Royal Manchester Children's Hospital, Central Manchester Foundation Trust, Manchester M13 9WL, UK

impaired, excepting a slight reduction in processing speed (Ebbink et al. 2012; Spiridigliozzi et al. 2013). Even in the two case reports with recorded white matter changes in early childhood, one was gaining clinical skills (Rohrbach et al. 2010) and while clinical decline was noted in the second case. This was related to both the expected myopathy and an additional peripheral neuropathy, rather than be central in origin (Burrow et al. 2010). Indeed, only recently have there been suggestions that IOPD patients may be at risk of a clinically significant sequelae from progressive central nervous system disease. The most prominent case thus far thus involved a 9-year-old IOPD patient whose observed intellectual decline was linked with extensive and progressive periventricular and subcortical white matter lesions (Ebbink et al. 2016). We report progressive white matter changes presenting in early childhood in a classical IOPD patient and their clinical impact, where extensive biochemical and genetic investigations have failed to show alternative causation to IOPD.

Methods

The genetic investigations were performed using a combination of Next Generation Sequencing (NGS) approaches. The first NGS analysis utilised a preselected vitamin and organic acid subpanels in an in-house panel of 226 genes involved with known metabolic pathways (Ghosh et al. 2017). Here DNA from a sample of blood was enriched by an Agilent SureSelect Custom Design target-enrichment kit (Agilent, Santa Clara, CA, USA) and sequenced with Illumina HiSeq 2500 (Illumina, Inc., San Diego, CA, USA). Subsequent sequence alignment, variant calling and annotation and filtering strategy were performed as reported previously from our laboratory (Ellingford et al. 2016). The second NGS approach was a targeted exome approach using genes selected based on both the 2015 consensus document for the definition of leukodystrophies and leukoencephalopathies (Vanderver et al. 2015) and those known to cause hereditary paraplegias (Hensiek et al. 2015). The hereditary paraplegias looked at were those with an autosomal recessive inheritance, presenting with a pure paraplegia or a complex presentation with documented leukodystrophy. As with the NGS panel the target exome used DNA derived from peripheral blood sampling which was enriched using Agilent SureSelectXT Focused Exome (Agilent, Santa Clara, CA, USA) and sequenced on the NextSeq500 (Illumina, Inc., San Diego, CA, USA). Variant calling using samtools v0.1.18, with hg19 human genome as a reference, and analysis performed using VarSeq®

(Golden Helix, Bozeman, MT, USA) to identify variants present in the genes of interest with an allele frequency <1% in control populations.

CSF glucose tetrasaccharide analysis by HPLC was performed on a sample snap frozen with liquid nitrogen at the bedside, using the methodology previously described (Prunty et al. 2015).

Patient and Results

The patient, part of an extended consanguineous family affected with IOPD, was initially noted to have hypertrophic cardiomyopathy on prenatal echo at 30 weeks' gestation. He was subsequently born spontaneously, prematurely at 33 + 4 weeks' gestation. On delivery, minimal cardiac hypertrophy was seen but no other clinical abnormalities identified. Confirmation of IOPD was via lymphocyte assay and genotyping. The later showing him to be homozygous for the familial c.2237G>A p.(Trp746*) mutation, a severe mutation (Beesley et al. 1998) associated with a CRIM Negative phenotype (Broomfield et al. 2016). Immunomodulation with four doses of rituximab (375 mg/M^2) and low dose methotrexate (2 doses of 0.4 mg/kg around the first six infusions) and subcutaneous immunoglobulin support was thus initiated with the onset of Myozyme 20 mg/kg weekly at 35 weeks' gestation. This dose of Myozyme was continued weekly for the first 3 months then given alternate weeks as per national protocol. No immediate acute complications were observed, with lymphocytic reconstitution occurring at 11 months of age. Clinical progress was good with normal developmental milestones achieved over the first 3 years of life with steady walking achieved at 16 months. No anti-Myozyme IgG antibodies have ever been detected.

However, at 3 years 10 months a change in gait was noted. On examination, there was increasing tightness initially in the left, then bilaterally in dorsiflexors and ultimately tight Achilles tendons. This was associated with hyperreflexia of the ankle reflexes but no other defects in peripheral neurology with proximal lower limb power remaining good and normal knee reflexes (see Fig. 1). This progressed over the course of the next year resulting in a loss of ambulation. An increase in dysarthria was noted 6 months after the lower limb signs, however audiology, cardiac and polysomnography were still unremarkable. One year on dysphagia has developed with aspiration seen on videofluoroscopy. The latest Wechsler Preschool and Primary Scale of Intelligence (WPPSI–IV)

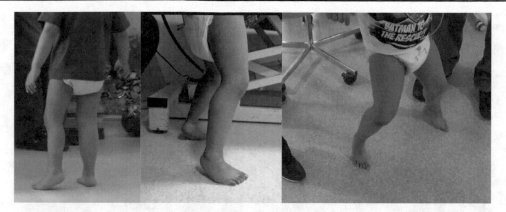

Fig. 1 Progression of distal spasticity in lower limb spasticity series, taken at 3 years 9 months to 4 years 4 months and 5 years

performed at 4 years 10 months, showed global severe impairment.

Given the increasingly distal lower limb spasticity, the history of prematurity and the consanguinity of the family, a central nervous system pathology was considered the most likely aetiology, possibly unrelated to the infantile onset Pompe disease. MRI brain at just over 4 years of age showed a predominately frontoparietal white matter involvement, initially mildly more extensive on the right than the left reflecting clinical symptomology. The subsequent imaging 6 months later showed progression of the changes but now included mild new bilateral involvement of the external capsules. Follow-up imaging also included single voxel MR Spectroscopy TE = 30 ms obtained from the region of the right basal ganglia and the left frontal deep white matter. Spectrum from the affected left frontal deep white matter was abnormal, with increased choline (Cho) and inositol (Ins) peaks, and reduced N-acetyl Aspartate peak, reflecting myelin and neuronal loss. MR Imaging findings are shown in Fig. 2.

Extensive biochemical, autoimmune and infective work up was initiated on the discovery of the white matter changes. Paired Plasma and CSF amino acids, lactates and glucose were all unremarkable as were CSF pterins, B6 and biogenic amine analysis. Similarly, acyl and plasma carnitines, plasma total homocysteine, cholesterol, plasma urate, VLCFAs, transferrin isoelectrofocusing, white cell enzymology and urinary profiling for purine and pyrimidine, bile acid, oligosaccharides and glycosaminoglycans. The only detectable biochemical abnormality was a CSF MTHF of 35 nmol/l (normal range 52–105), though plasma and red cell folate levels were within the normal range. The patient has been subsequently supplemented with oral calcium folinate at 15 mg/day without discernible response. Glucose tetrasaccharide (Glc4) in CSF was undetectable by HPLC analysis. The infective work up showed negative plasma and CSF PCR for VZZ, HSV, enterovirus and prior JC polyomavirus (JCV) infection. Immunological work up included normal total immunoglobulin, ANA, pANCA levels with anti-phospholipid antibodies being absent. Vitamin E and copper, the biochemical causes of spasticity not already covered in the biochemical white matter screen were also found to be normal.

Initial genetic profiling concentrated on known causes of low CSF folate and showed no pathogenic variants in FOLR1, MTHFR, SLC46A1, DHFR, and indeed only two variants of unknown significance in BCKDHD and PCCA both of which could be excluded as pathogenic based on the normal biochemistry. Similarly blood mitochondrial DNA analysis for common point mutations, deletions and duplications was normal. Subsequent analysis using the targeted exome revealed eight variants of unknown significance in eight genes. For the full list of genes selected and coverage please see Appendix, all the primary leukodystrophies, as classified by a recent European consensus group (Vanderver et al. 2015), had good coverage with none of the eight variants identified are predicted to be pathogenic (Richards et al. 2015).

Discussion

The case is the youngest treated IOPD patient who has demonstrated centrally mediated neurological regression. Given the consanguineous background, extensive investigation was attempted to ensure no secondary disease was

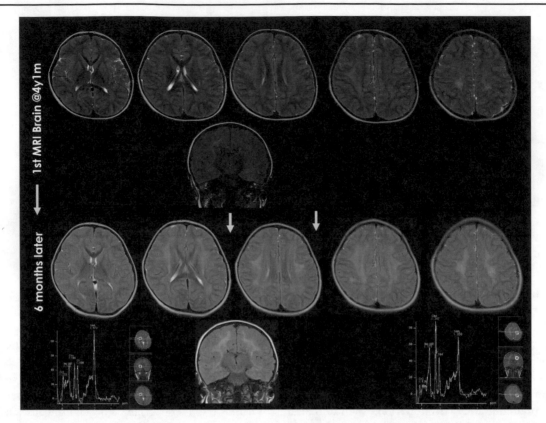

Fig. 2 MRI brain and MR spectroscopy findings. First row: initial MRI brain at 4 years. Five axial T2 images from the level of the internal capsules to the level of the centrum semiovale, and a coronal FLAIR image through the corona radiata. These demonstrate bilateral white matter changes with frontoparietal predominance involving the periventricular, deep and subcortical white matter with sparing of the U-fibres and internal capsules. In the lower row, the corresponding images to first row are displayed taken at 4 years 7 months. These demonstrate the progression of the white matter changes, which now

also includes new mild bilateral involvement of the external capsules. The single voxel MR spectroscopy at the age of 4 years 7 month, on the left obtained from the right basal ganglia, and on the right from the affected left frontal deep white matter. Apart from an increased Myoinositol (Ins) peak, the main metabolites spectrum from the right basal ganglia is within normal limits for the patient's age. The spectrum from the affected left frontal deep white matter is abnormal with increased Choline (Cho) and Ins peaks, and reduced NAA peak, reflecting myelin and neuronal loss

present, both to rule out a second treatable pathology and or identify potential targets for wider family screening. The only abnormal biochemical finding was a low CSF folate, though the level was not suggestive of a primary disorder of folate metabolism. Indeed, the subsequent sequencing of the genes involved in folate metabolism failed to show primary defect nor were any mitochondrial DNA point mutations, duplications or deletions defined in blood. The level of the folate was not suggestive of a primary defect and may well, given the extensive pathological cascades established in Pompe, reflect ongoing oxidative stress (Aylett et al. 2013). The likelihood of the leukodystrophy being driven by a reduction in CSF Methyltetrahydrofolate levels is further reduced by the lack of response to calcium folinate supplementation. There were no obvious infective or immunological triggers seen with JCV infection

specifically investigated, given its known association with progressive multifocal leukoencephalopathy post rituximab utilisation (Jelcic et al. 2015).

The lack of an alternative diagnosis despite extensive the biochemical and genetic work up would support the inference that, the progressive white matter disease was secondary to the patient's IOPD. Radiological comparison of this case to those previously documented would also seem to support this supposition. In total, there are currently eight reported IOPD patients on ERT with MRI changes (Burrow et al. 2010; Chien et al. 2006; Ebbink et al. 2016; Rohrbach et al. 2010). The radiology in these cases is very similar to this case, with all patients showing a periventricular white matter involvement with apparent sparing of the U fibres. Given the extent of the white matter disease in this patient, it was somewhat surprising to see sparing of the internal capsule, however myelination was observed in the internal capsule in all five of the case series of Chien et al., albeit at a slightly later age than expected (Chien et al. 2006). In the oldest patient, there was again periventricular involvement and subcortical white matter involvement with subcortical predominance (Ebbink et al. 2016). Both the Ebbink et al. case and the patient here had involvement of the corticospinal tracts including the internal capsule, though Ebbink et al. reported no overt clinical sequelae unlike this case.

Mechanistically the potential for central neurological involvement in IOPD has been frequently postulated (Burrow et al. 2010; Chen et al. 2004; Rohrbach et al. 2010). Historical autopsies clearly demonstrate the presence of widespread glycogen deposition in the brain (Gambetti et al. 1971; Mancall et al. 1965; Martin et al. 1973; Shotelersuk et al. 2002). Typically, the autopsies show greatest neuronal glycogen accumulation in the cranial motor nuclei and cerebellar nuclei (Mancall et al. 1965; Martin et al. 1973) with minimal build up in the cerebral cortex (Mancall et al. 1965; Martin et al. 1973; Teng et al. 2004). However, despite limited glycogen deposition the in the cortex, past autopsies have shown both neuronal loss (Mancall et al. 1965) and extensive gliosis. Indeed, in IOPD autopsies glial cell accumulation appears to be greatest in the white matter (Gambetti et al. 1971; Martin et al. 1973). This process of neuronal loss and gliosis would be supported by the spectroscopic findings in this case and the limited previous spectroscopic data (Burrow et al. 2010; Chien et al. 2006) where low NAA/creatinine ratios, suggesting neuronal loss, and raised Choline/creatinine ratio indicative of either demyelination or gliosis have been noted.

Given their pivotal role in CNS myelination (Bercury and Macklin 2015), it is always important to consider the role of oligodendrocytes in any white matter abnormality, especially given that in IOPD, oligodendritic accumulate of glycogen outweighs that of other glial cells (Gambetti et al. 1971). For although absolute oligodendrocyte numbers appear not to be altered In IOPD (Gambetti et al. 1971; Mancall et al. 1965), little is known about the potential impact of glycogen accumulation on oligodendrocyte function. However, given the impact of α-glucosidase has on mTOR regulation (Lim et al. 2017) and the importance of mTOR has on oligodendrocyte differentiation (Bercury et al. 2014), the potential for oligodendrocyte dysfunction in IOPD seems a worthwhile avenue worthy of further investigation.

Given that glycogen accumulation is the pivotal pathological determinant in the subcellular cascades (Lim et al. 2014), it interesting to note that the patients with the most extensive radiological neurological involvement reported thus far, have demonstrated or would be predicted to show the lowest enzymatic activity. Thus case 1, the most severely affected of the series of Chien et al. (2006), had the lowest fibroblast, while the both the patient reported here and that in the case of Rohrbach et al. (2010), have genotypes predictive of no functional protein production. It may thus be the central nervous system involvement in part underlies the seemingly worse outcome in CRIM negative patients (Kishnani et al. 2010), with increasing suggestions that the poor outcome may not always be antibody mediated (Broomfield et al. 2016). The paradigm being that even minimal increases in glycogen clearance, affected by minimally functioning α-glucosidase results in milder CNS disease. This seems to be born out given the variability in the amount of glycogen found in the CNS in children diagnosed in early childhood (Martini et al. 2001; Martin et al. 1976).

In conclusion, this is the earliest case of apparent progressive CNS disease documented thus far in the classical onset IOPD population, where extensive investigation has failed to find an alternative causation. It adds to the growing evidence that the CNS accumulation of glycogen in classical onset IOPD cases may not be as benign as previously considered and may indicate the need for greater surveillance of the central nervous system in the IOPD population from an early age. For although thus far the clear majority of IOPD patients have no apparent manifestations of progressive white matter involvement, CNS involvement should at least be considered in IOPD who are showing increasing functional loss, whatever their age.

Synopsis

Some patients with the classical variant of infantile onset Pompe disease run the risk of an early childhood onset progressive white matter involvement.

Details of the Contributions of Individual Authors

Dr. Broomfield conceived and was the main author of the manuscript.

Miss Fletcher: Helped collect data and has critically reviewed the manuscript.

Miss Hensman: Helped collect data and has critically reviewed the manuscript.

Mr. Wright: Both performed and analysed the data of the NGS investigations. He also critically reviewed the manuscript.

Miss Prunty performed the CSF HPLS tetrasaccharide assay and critically reviewed the manuscript.

Dr. Pavaine reviewed and selected the neuroimaging and critically reviewed the manuscript.

Dr. Jones helped collect data and conception of the manuscript and has reviewed the manuscript.

Corresponding Author

Dr. A Broomfield

Competing Interest Statement

Dr. Broomfield and Dr. Jones have both received travel funding, teaching Honoria from and have done consultancy for Sanofi-Genzyme. The other authors have no conflict of interest of note.

Details of Funding

No funding was involved in this study and the authors confirm that the content of the article has not been influenced by the sponsors.

Details of Ethics Approval

Not applicable, given the nature of this case report.

A Patient Consent Statement

Parental consent for the use of the images has been granted.

Documentation of Approval from the Institutional Committee for Care and Use of Laboratory Animals

Not applicable given the nature of this case report.

Appendix

Genes examined by NGS targeted panel approach:

ABCD4, ACSF3, AMN, AUH, BCKDHA, BTD, CD320, CUBN, DBT, DHFR, DHFRL1, DNAJC19, FOLR1, FLOR2, FOLR3, FTCD, GIF, HCFC1, HLCS, IVD, LMBRD1, MCCC1, MCCC2, MCEE, MMAA, MMAB, MMACHC, MTHFD1, MTHFR, MTR, MTRR, MUT, OPA3, PCCA, PCCB, PPMIK, SERAC1, SLC19A3, SCL46A1, SLC52A1, SLC52A2, SLC5A3, SCULA2, SUCLG1, TAZ, TCN1, TCN2, TMEM70.

Unclassified variants identified through screening were the BCKDHD c.-4G>C heterozygote and PCCA C.1236A>G p.(Pro421Pro) het.

Genes examined using NGS targeted exome approach:

ACOX1, ACP5, AIMP1, ATN1, ATP7B, BCAP31, CGA, CLCN2, CLCN7, COL4A1, COL4A2, CSF1R, CTC1, DARS, DARS2, DCAF17, EARS2, EIF2B1, EIF2B2, EIF2B3, EIF2B4, EIF2B5,ERCC2, ERCC3, ERCC5, ERCC6, ERCC8, FA2H, FAM126A, FARS2, FHL1, FHL2, FKRP, FKTN, GAN, GBE1, GFAP, GJA1, GJC2, GPR56, GTF2H5, HSD17B4, HSPD1, HTRA1, JAM3, LAMA2, LARGE, LMNB1, MAGT1, MARS2, MLC1, MPLKIP, NDUFS1, NOTCH3, NPC1, NPC2, NUBPL, OCLN, OCRL, OSTM1, PEX1,PEX2,PEX3, PEX5,PEX6, PEX7, PEX10, PEX11B, PEX12, PEX13, PEX14, PEX16, PEX19, PEX26, PLP1, PMM2, POLD1, POLR1C, POLR3A, POLR3B, POMGNT1, POMT1, POMT2.

RNASET2, SLC16A2, SLC17A5, SLC25A12, SLC7A2, SPG5A, SPG7, SPG11, SPG15, SPG18, SPG26, SPG35, PG53, TREM2, TUBB4A, TYROBP, ZFYVE26.

Unclassified variants identified using NGS targeted exome approach:

NM_025000.3 DCAF17 c.1030T>C p.(Trp344Arg) het

NM_004366.5 CLCN2 c.1930C>T p.(Arg644Cys) het

NM_003630.2 PEX3 c.161G>A p.(Arg54Gln) het

NM_001940.3 ATN1 c.1500_1508delGCAGCAGCA p.(Gln500_Gln502del) het

NM_000053.3 ATP7B c.442C>T p.(Arg148Trp) het

NM_013382.5 POMT2 c.2223A>G p.(=) het

NM_025137.3 SPG11 c.3146-4C>A het

NM_152415.2 SPG53 c.834A.G het

Gene	% Coverage 20X	Gene	% Coverage 20X	Gene	% Coverage 20X
ACOX1	99.21	FKRP	100.00	PEX13	99.76
ACP5	100.00	FKTN	89.70	PEX14	100.00
AIMP1	95.27	GAN	97.29	PEX16	91.67
ATN1	99.66	GBE1	98.70	PEX19	99.45
ATP7B	98.34	GFAP	99.86	PEX2	100.00
BCAP31	59.10	GJA1	15.48	PEX26	100.00
CGA	100.00	GJC2	99.70	PEX3	100.00
CLCN2	100.00	GPR56	100.00	PEX5	100.00
CLCN7	100.00	GTF2H5	85.32	PEX6	99.81
COL4A1	98.73	HSD17B4	90.47	PEX7	100.00
COL4A2	99.82	HSPD1	24.58	PLP1	84.96
CSF1R	99.68	HTRA1	99.51	PMM2	98.04
CTC1	99.27	JAM3	100.00	POLD1	99.72
DARS	94.11	LAMA2	97.72	POLR1C	97.60
DARS2	98.38	LARGE	100.00	POLR3A	98.36
DCAF17	96.69	LMNB1	97.64	POLR3B	95.37
EARS2	98.87	MAGT1	71.95	POMGNT1	100.00
EIF2B1	100.00	MARS2	100.00	POMT1	98.92
EIF2B2	99.46	MLC1	100.00	POMT2	99.51
EIF2B3	99.46	MPLKIP	99.55	RARS	91.00
EIF2B4	99.90	NDUFS1	98.59	RNASET2	90.60
EIF2B5	100.00	NOTCH3	99.83	SLC16A2	90.74
ERCC2	99.57	NPC1	98.25	SLC17A5	93.60
ERCC3	98.07	NPC2	100.00	SLC25A12	96.35
ERCC5	95.65	NUBPL	87.84	SLC7A2	96.77
ERCC6	97.95	OCLN	37.50	SPG11	91.76
ERCC8	89.66	OCRL	92.60	TREM2	100.00
FA2H	100.00	OSTM1	82.40	TUBB4A	88.73
FAM126A	98.06	PEX1	95.55	TYROBP	99.77
FARS2	100.00	PEX10	100.00	ZFYVE26	98.57
FHL1	83.54	PEX11B	96.28	Grand Total	95.95
FHL2	100.00	PEX12	99.19		

References

Aylett SB, Neergheen V, Hargreaves IP, Eaton S, Land JM, Rahman S, Heales SJ (2013) Levels of 5-methyltetrahydrofolate and ascorbic acid in cerebrospinal fluid are correlated: implications for the accelerated degradation of folate by reactive oxygen species. Neurochem Int 63:750–755

Beesley CE, Child AH, Yacoub MH (1998) The identification of five novel mutations in the lysosomal acid a-(1-4) glucosidase gene from patients with glycogen storage disease type II. Mutations in brief no. 134. Online. Hum Mutat 11:413

Bercury KK, Dai J, Sachs HH, Ahrendsen JT, Wood TL, Macklin WB (2014) Conditional ablation of raptor or rictor has differential impact on oligodendrocyte differentiation and CNS myelination. J Neurosci 34:4466–4480

Bercury KK, Macklin WB (2015) Dynamics and mechanisms of CNS myelination. Dev Cell 32:447–458

Broomfield A, Fletcher J, Davison J et al (2016) Response of 33 UK patients with infantile-onset Pompe disease to enzyme replacement therapy. J Inherit Metab Dis 39:261–271

Burrow TA, Bailey LA, Kinnett DG, Hopkin RJ (2010) Acute progression of neuromuscular findings in infantile Pompe disease. Pediatr Neurol 42:455–458

Byrne BJ, Kishnani PS, Case LE, Merlini L, Muller-Felber W, Prasad S, van der Ploeg A (2011) Pompe disease: design, methodology, and early findings from the Pompe Registry. Mol Genet Metab 103:1–11

Chen CP, Lin SP, Tzen CY, Tsai FJ, Hwu WL, Wang W (2004) Detection of a homozygous D645E mutation of the acid alpha-glucosidase gene and glycogen deposition in tissues in a second-trimester fetus with infantile glycogen storage disease type II. Prenat Diagn 24:231–232

Chien YH, Lee NC, Peng SF, Hwu WL (2006) Brain development in infantile-onset Pompe disease treated by enzyme replacement therapy. Pediatr Res 60:349–352

Ebbink BJ, Aarsen FK, van Gelder CM et al (2012) Cognitive outcome of patients with classic infantile Pompe disease receiving enzyme therapy. Neurology 78:1512–1518

Ebbink BJ, Poelman E, Plug I, Lequin MH, van Doorn PA, Aarsen FK, van der Ploeg AT, van den Hout JMP (2016) Cognitive decline in classic infantile Pompe disease: an underacknowledged challenge. Neurology 86:1260–1261

Ellingford JM, Barton S, Bhaskar S et al (2016) Molecular findings from 537 individuals with inherited retinal disease. J Med Genet 53:761–767

Gambetti P, DiMauro S, Baker L (1971) Nervous system in Pompe's disease. Ultrastructure and biochemistry. J Neuropathol Exp Neurol 30:412–430

Ghosh A, Schlecht H, Heptinsall LE et al (2017) Diagnosing childhood-onset inborn errors of metabolism by next-generation. doi:10.1136/archdischild-2017-312737

Hensiek A, Kirker S, Reid E (2015) Diagnosis, investigation and management of hereditary spastic paraplegias in the era of next-generation sequencing. J Neurol 262:1601–1612

Hers HG (1963) Alpha-Glucosidase deficiency in generalized glycogenstorage disease (Pompe's disease). Biochem J 86:11–16

Jelcic I, Jelcic I, Faigle W, Sospedra M, Martin R (2015) Immunology of progressive multifocal leukoencephalopathy. J Neurovirol 21:614–622

Kishnani PS, Goldenberg PC, DeArmey SL et al (2010) Cross-reactive immunologic material status affects treatment outcomes in Pompe disease infants. Mol Genet Metab 99:26–33

Lim JA, Li L, Raben N (2014) Pompe disease: from pathophysiology to therapy and back again. Front Aging Neurosci 6:177

Lim JA, Li L, Shirihai OS, Trudeau KM, Puertollano R, Raben N (2017) Modulation of mTOR signaling as a strategy for the treatment of Pompe disease. EMBO Mol Med 9:353–370

Mancall EL, Aponte GE, Berry RG (1965) Pompe's disease (diffuse Glycogenosis) with neuronal storage. J Neuropathol Exp Neurol 24:85–96

Martin JJ, De Barsy T, De S, Leroy JG, Palladini G (1976) Acid maltase deficiency in non-identical adult twins. A morphological and biochemical study. J Neurol 213:105–118

Martin JJ, de Barsy T, van Hoof F, Palladini G (1973) Pompe's disease: an inborn lysosomal disorder with storage of glycogen. A study of brain and striated muscle. Acta Neuropathol 23:229–244

Martini C, Ciana G, Benettoni A, Katouzian F, Severini GM, Bussani R, Bembi B (2001) Intractable fever and cortical neuronal glycogen storage in glycogenosis type 2. Neurology 57:906–908

Prunty H, Man WC, Carey T, Lukovic B, Heales S (2015) Improved method for the analysis of urinary glucose tetrasaccharide (Glc4) by high pressure liquid chromatography (HPLC). Mol Genet Metab 114:S97–S97

Richards S, Aziz N, Bale S et al (2015) Standards and guidelines for the interpretation of sequence variants: a joint consensus recommendation of the American College of Medical Genetics and Genomics and the Association for Molecular Pathology. Genet Med 17:405–424

Rohrbach M, Klein A, Kohli-Wiesner A et al (2010) CRIM-negative infantile Pompe disease: 42-month treatment outcome. J Inherit Metab Dis 33:751–757

Shotelersuk V, Shuangshoti S, Chotivitayatarakorn P et al (2002) Clinical, pathological, and electron microscopic findings in two Thai children with Pompe disease. J Med Assoc Thail 85(Suppl 1):S271–S279

Spiridigliozzi GA, Heller JH, Kishnani PS et al (2013) Cognitive outcome of patients with classic infantile Pompe disease receiving enzyme therapy. Neurology 80:1173

Teng YT, Su WJ, Hou JW, Huang SF (2004) Infantile-onset glycogen storage disease type II (Pompe disease): report of a case with genetic diagnosis and pathological findings. Chang Gung Med J 27:379–384

van den Hout HM, Hop W, van Diggelen OP et al (2003) The natural course of infantile Pompe's disease: 20 original cases compared with 133 cases from the literature. Pediatrics 112:332–340

Vanderver A, Prust M, Tonduti D et al (2015) Case definition and classification of leukodystrophies and leukoencephalopathies. Mol Genet Metab 114:494–500

JIMD Reports
DOI 10.1007/8904_2017_40

RESEARCH REPORT

Four Years' Experience in the Diagnosis of Very Long-Chain Acyl-CoA Dehydrogenase Deficiency in Infants Detected in Three Spanish Newborn Screening Centers

B. Merinero · P. Alcaide · E. Martín-Hernández ·
A. Morais · M. T. García-Silva · P. Quijada-Fraile ·
C. Pedrón-Giner · E. Dulin · R. Yahyaoui ·
J. M. Egea · A. Belanger-Quintana · J. Blasco-Alonso ·
M. L. Fernandez Ruano · B. Besga · I. Ferrer-López ·
F. Leal · M. Ugarte · P. Ruiz-Sala · B. Pérez ·
C. Pérez-Cerdá

Received: 13 March 2017 / Revised: 08 June 2017 / Accepted: 15 June 2017 / Published online: 29 July 2017
© SSIEM and Springer-Verlag Berlin Heidelberg 2017

Abstract Identification of very long-chain acyl-CoA dehydrogenase deficiency is possible in the expanded newborn screening (NBS) due to the increase in tetradecenoylcarnitine (C14:1) and in the C14:1/C2, C14:1/C16, C14:1/C12:1 ratios detected in dried blood spots. Nevertheless, different confirmatory tests must be performed to confirm the final diagnosis. We have revised the NBS results and the results of the confirmatory tests (plasma acylcarnitine profiles, molecular findings, and lymphocytes VLCAD activity) for 36 cases detected in three Spanish NBS centers during 4 years, correlating these with the clinical outcome and treatment. Our aim was to distinguish unambiguously true cases from disease carriers in order to obtain useful

diagnostic information for clinicians that can be applied in the follow-up of neonates identified by NBS.

Increases in C14:1 and of the different ratios, the presence of two pathogenic mutations, and deficient enzyme activity in lymphocytes ($<12\%$ of the intra-assay control) identified 12 true-positive cases. These cases were given nutritional therapy and all of them are asymptomatic, except one. Seventeen individuals were considered disease carriers based on the mild increase in plasma C14:1, in conjunction with the presence of only one mutation and/or intermediate residual activity (18–57%). In addition, seven cases were classified as false positives, with normal biochemical parameters and no mutations in the exonic region of *ACADVL*. All these carriers and the false positive cases remained asymptomatic. The combined evaluation of the acylcarnitine profiles, genetic results, and residual enzyme

Communicated by: Piero Rinaldo, MD, PhD

B. Merinero (✉) · P. Alcaide · I. Ferrer-López · F. Leal · M. Ugarte ·
P. Ruiz-Sala · B. Pérez · C. Pérez-Cerdá
Centro de Diagnóstico de Enfermedades Moleculares, Centro de
Biología Molecular-SO UAM-CSIC, Universidad Autónoma de
Madrid, Centro de Investigación Biomédica en Red de Enfermedades
Raras (CIBERER), IdiPAZ, Madrid, Spain
e-mail: bmerinero@cbm.csic.es

E. Martín-Hernández · M.T. García-Silva · P. Quijada-Fraile
Departamento de Pediatría, Unidad de Enfermedades Mitocondriales-
Metabólicas Hereditarias, Hospital Universitario Doce de Octubre,
Universidad Complutense de Madrid, CIBERER, Madrid, Spain

A. Morais
Unidad de Nutrición Infantil y Enfermedades Metabólicas, Hospital
Universitario Infantil La Paz, Madrid, Spain

C. Pedrón-Giner
Sección de Gastroenterología y Nutrición, Hospital Infantil
Universitario Niño Jesús, Madrid, Spain

E. Dulin · M.L. Fernandez Ruano · B. Besga
Laboratorio de Cribado Neonatal, Hospital General Universitario
Gregorio Marañón, Madrid, Spain

R. Yahyaoui
Laboratorio de Metabolopatías, Hospital Regional de Málaga, Instituto
de Investigación Biomédica de Málaga (IBIMA), Málaga, Spain

J.M. Egea
Centro de Bioquímica y Genética Clínica, Unidad de Metabolopatías,
Hospital General Universitario Virgen de la Arrixaca, Murcia, Spain

A. Belanger-Quintana
Unidad de Enfermedades Metabólicas, Servicio de Pediatría, Hospital
Universitario Ramón y Cajal, Madrid, Spain

J. Blasco-Alonso
Sección de Gastroenterología y Nutrición Pediátrica, Hospital
Regional de Málaga, Málaga, Spain

activities have proven useful to definitively classify individuals with suspected VLCAD deficiency into true-positive cases and carriers, and to decide which cases need treatment.

Introduction

Very long-chain acyl-CoA dehydrogenase (VLCAD) is a membrane-bound mitochondrial enzyme involved in the ß-oxidation of long-chain fatty acids that is encoded by *ACADVL*. Patients with VLCAD deficiency (VLCADD; MIM 201475) have a varied clinical phenotype: a severe early-onset form that is associated with a high incidence of cardiomyopathy and high mortality; an intermediate form with childhood onset that is usually associated with hypoketotic hypoglycemia, hepatopathy, and a more favorable outcome; and an adult-onset, myopathic form with isolated skeletal muscle involvement, rhabdomyolysis, and myoglobinuria after exercise or fasting (Andresen et al. 1999; Merinero et al. 1999). The accumulation of tetradecenoylcarnitine (C14:1) in plasma is a biomarker of this disease, and some correlations between genotype and phenotype have been established. Thus, patients with null mutations in *ACADVL* that provoke a loss of activity have more severe symptoms than those that retain some residual activity (Andresen et al. 1999).

The determination of acylcarnitines (AC) in dried blood spots (DBS) by tandem mass spectrometry (MS/MS) has enabled VLCADD to be identified in presymptomatic newborns through the elevation of its primary marker C14:1, and of the C14:1/C2, C14:1/C16 and C14:1/C12:1 ratios (Merritt et al. 2014). Early disease detection by newborn screening (NBS) is absolutely essential to achieve a more favorable clinical outcome and indeed, it helps to significantly reduce disease mortality and morbidity (Arnold et al. 2009; Spiekerkoetter et al. 2009). Since its introduction into NBS programs, the number of cases of VLCADD detected has increased, reaching an estimated prevalence of 1:31,500–50,000 (Boneh et al. 2006; Spiekerkoetter et al. 2010). This increase could be explained by the detection of either milder phenotypes or asymptomatic individuals, even by the identification of false-positives. In fact, the mild accumulation of long-chain AC can be observed in healthy children due to the activation of mitochondrial fatty acid oxidation during catabolism in the first days of life (Boneh et al. 2006). Thus, each newborn with a suggestive VLCADD AC profile requires further confirmatory diagnosis (ter Veld et al. 2009).

Molecular and/or enzyme assays have been recommended as second-level testing for VLCADD (Browning et al. 2005). However, genetic analysis alone may be inconclusive in predicting the risk of future metabolic decompensation as new nucleotide variants of unknown clinical

significance are often identified (Coughlin and Ficicioglu 2010). Besides, as there is considerable molecular heterogeneity in VLCADD, genotyping is not always a swift and cost-effective confirmatory diagnostic technique (ter Veld et al. 2009). Despite the use of different tests, the confirmation of a VLCADD diagnosis identified in NBS still requires several rounds of discussion (Pena et al. 2016).

In this study we have revised the NBS results, the diagnostic evaluation through plasma AC profiles, the molecular findings and lymphocyte VLCAD activity, as well as the clinical outcome and treatment of 36 cases detected over 4 years in three Spanish NBS centers. The aim of the study was to unambiguously distinguish true VLCADD cases from carriers of the disease and from false-positive cases, and to provide useful diagnostic information to clinicians in the follow-up of NBS identified neonates.

Materials and Methods

Patients

A retrospective analysis was performed on the clinical evaluation and results of confirmatory tests carried out on 36 neonates with suspected VLCADD that were detected by MS/MS between April 2011 and December 2015 among 619,906 newborns in three Spanish screening centers (Madrid, Eastern Andalucía and Murcia). Each center had previously independently determined its internal NBS 99.5 percentile cut-off levels and the criteria for a positive screen of newborns at 48–72 h of life. Cut-offs for C14:1 ranged from 0.27 to 0.50 μmol/L, and for C14:1/C2 from 0.015 to 0.030, C14:1/C16 from 0.087 to 0.14 and/or of C14:1/C12:1 from 7 to 7.3.

The data for all cases were analyzed using the current Region 4 VLCADD general single post-analytical tool. The Region 4 Stork (R4S) Collaborative Project is a database developed for newborn screening quality improvement (Hall et al. 2014). This tool calculates predictive score for VLCADD based on newborn screening analytes including C14:1, C14, C14:2, C16:1, C16OH, C12, C12:1 and ratios thereof. A score of ≥ 100 is "very likely" to be VLCADD, >50–100 is "likely" to be VLCADD, ≥ 10–50 is "possibly" VLCADD, and <10 "not informative".

The identified cases were remitted to their clinical reference units for confirmation of VLCADD between 7 and 20 days post-partum. In all cases the confirmatory tests involved measuring the plasma AC levels, the organic acids in urine and a thorough molecular analysis of *ACADVL*. In some selected cases, namely those with two mutations or those with only one variant of unknown clinical significance, VLCAD enzyme activity in lymphocytes was

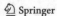

assessed by MS/MS. Parents signed a written informed consent for the mutation analysis and/or the assessment of enzyme activity.

Biochemical Analysis

Acylcarnitines were analyzed in plasma as described previously (Ferrer et al. 2007). Organic acids were determined by GC/MS as trimethylsilyl derivatives after urease treatment and ethyl acetate liquid–liquid extraction without oxymation.

VLCAD Enzyme Activity in Lymphocytes

The method used to assess VLCAD activity is based on the oxidation of palmitoyl-CoA (C16:0-CoA) in the presence of the electron acceptor, ferrocenium hexafluorophosphate ($FcPF_6$), essentially as described for MCAD activity (Tajima et al. 2005). Lymphocytes were isolated from whole blood (3–5 mL) using Histopaque (Sigma-Aldrich, Deisenhofen, Germany) and the resulting pellet was frozen before use. The lymphocytes were resuspended in a buffer containing 125 mmol/L KH_2PO_4, 1 mmol/L EDTA and 9% Triton X-100, and they were then sonicated twice for 5 min, kept on ice for 30 min and finally, centrifuged at 12,000 rpm for 10 min. The reaction mixtures contained 5 mmol/L C16:0-CoA, 4 mmol/L $FcFP_6$, in a final volume of 100 μL.

The analysis of C16:0-CoA and the 2-hexadecenoyl-CoA (C16:1-CoA) and 3-hydroxyhexadecanoyl-CoA (C16OH-CoA) reaction products was performed by LC-MS/MS (1100 Agilent Series HPLC, Santa Clara, California, USA), with the apparatus coupled to an Applied Biosystems API 2000 QTrap (Carlsbad, California, USA). A 5 μL aliquot of each sample was injected onto a Symmetry C18 column (100 mm × 2.1 mm, particle size 3.5 μm, Waters) and the mobile phase consisted of 10 mmol/L ammonium acetate in a mixture of H_2O:ACN (45:55). The flow rate was 200 μL/min, and the run time was 20 min. Acyl-CoAs were analyzed in positive multiple reaction monitoring (MRM) mode, with MRM transitions of 1,006 → 499 for C16:0-CoA, 1,004 → 497 for C16:1-CoA and 1,022 → 515 for standard C16OH-CoA. Quantification was based on the peak area [sum of products areas/(sum of substrate + products areas) ratio], with the initial amount of C16:0-CoA substrate set to 20 nmol (ter Veld et al. 2009). Proteins were quantified by the Lowry method prior to adding Triton X-100.

Product formation was shown to be linear for up to 15 min and proportional to the amount of protein added in the range of 20–200 μg, with a correlation coefficient of $r^2 = 0.99$. The limit of C16:1-CoA or C16OH-CoA detection (signal/noise >3) was estimated to be 0.015 nmol/min/mg protein. The intra-day reproducibility of VLCAD activity was calculated in one control sample, realizing multiple replicates that revealed an imprecision coefficient of 1.8%, indicative of satisfactory reproducibility in the analysis.

Mutation Analysis

Genotypes were analyzed by exon sequencing of the *ACADVL* locus using conventional Sanger sequencing or massive parallel sequencing. Massive parallel sequencing was done using a targeted customized panel to capture the exome of 120 genes involved in metabolic disorders (Nextera Nature Capture, Illumina, San Diego, California, USA: the list of genes included can be sent upon request). The mean depth of coverage was 292× (99.9%) for the *ACADVL* gene. Mutations are named according to the HGVS nomenclature (http://www.hgvs.org/mutnomen), using the RefSeq number NM_000018.3. New single nucleotide variants (SNVs) were analyzed using Alamut Visual Software to predict their pathogenic effect and all variant changes were confirmed by Sanger sequencing in parental samples.

Clinical Parameters

A clinical questionnaire was sent to the referring physicians to collect data regarding the neonatal screening, family origin, consanguinity, pregnancy and delivery, neonatal complications, nutritional treatment (low-LCT diet, MCT, and/or carnitine supplementation), metabolic decompensation, and clinical evaluation (weight, height and head circumference parameters, routine laboratory findings, neurological and cardiological examinations).

Statistical Analysis

A non-parametric Mann–Whitney U-test (two-tailed) was used to assess the significance of the differences in AC levels between the groups, with a p value <0.05 considered significant.

Results

Newborn Screening

Fifteen cases presented a significant elevation of C14:1 (1.02–7.55 μmol/L), as well as the enhanced C14:1/C2 and C14:1/C16 ratios in DBS (P1–P10, P13–P17: Tables 1 and 2). Ratio C14:1/C12:1 was also found elevated in some of them (P1, P3, P4, P5, P7, P8, P10). The remaining individuals had elevated C14:1 ranging from 0.44 to 0.93 μmol/L and/or C12, C12:1, C14, C14:2 (data not

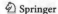

Table 1 Clinical, biochemical, and molecular findings in VLCADD cases identified by NBS with bi-allelic mutations in *ACADVL*

	DBS (NBS) (48 h)				Plasma (confirmatory test)								
	C14:1 (µmol/L)	C14:1/ C2	C14:1/ C16	C14:1/ C12:1	C14:1 (µmol/L)	C14:1/ C2	C14:1/ C16	C14:1/ C12:1	Maternal allele	Paternal allele	VLCAD activity[a] (LF) (%)	Therapy[b]	Age/clinical outcome[c]
					<1 month >1 month[e]	<1 month >1 month[e]	<1 month >1 month[e]	<1 month >1 month[e]					
NR[d]	<0.27–0.50	<0.015–0.030	<0.037–0.140	<7–7.3	<0.17 / <0.17	<0.023 / <0.012	<1.27 / <2.39	<5.69 / <2.65					
ID													
P1	7.55	0.29	1.05	9.7	1.69	0.28	8.9	33.8	**c.761G>A (p.Gly254Asp)**	c.761G>A (p.Gly254Asp)	1.5	LMC	5.5 years/ Asymp
P2	5.02	0.19	0.51	5.8	2.74	0.28	4.9	7.2	**c.1174G>C (p.Val392Leu)**	**c.1752-2_1755del6 (p.?)**	2.8	LM	18 months/ Asymp
P3	4.45[f]	0.77[f]	0.38[f]	49.4[f]	1.70[e]	0.74[e]	2.0[e]	56.7[e]	c.643T>C (p.Cys215Arg)	c.643T>C (p.Cys215Arg)	BLD	LMC	3 years/MD (n:8), Hep, Myo; HC
P4	4.16	0.18	0.53	10.4	0.77	0.09	4.8	15.4	c.848T>C (p.Val283Ala)	**c.996delT (p.Ala333Profs*20)**	NS	M	4.5 years/ Asymp
P5	3.37	0.09	0.48	8.3	3.01	0.44	4.9	21.5	[c.1097G>A; c.1844G>A] (p.Arg366His; p.Arg615Gln)	[c.1097G>A; c.1844G>A] (p.Arg366His; p.Arg615Gln)	1.1	LC	14 months/ PST; I (15 days) Asymp
P6	3.30	0.11	0.44	4.5	0.87	0.11	3.0	4.4	c.848T>C (p.Val283Ala)	c.848T>C (p.Val283Ala)	8.8	LMC	3 years/ Asymp
P7	2.78	0.20	1.07	15.4	1.58	0.20	11.3	39.5	c.848T>C (p.Val283Ala)	c.685C>T (p.Arg229Ter)	2.7	LMC	5.5 years/ Asymp
P8	2.65	0.20	0.74	12.0	1.73	0.37	6.0	19.2	c.848T>C/c.685C>T (p.Val283Ala/p.Arg229Ter)		9.9	LMC	4.5 years/ Asymp
P9[g]	1.36	0.10	1.07	3.8	0.55	0.07	5.0	5.5	**c.1220G>C (p.Gly407Ala)**	c.848T>C (p.Val283Ala)	11.8	M	5 years/ Asymp
P10	1.25	0.10	0.30	11.4	0.79	0.10	7.2	26.3	c.520G>A (p.Val174Met)	[c.1097G>A; c.1844G>A] (p.Arg366His; p.Arg615Gln)	3.7	LMC	5.5 years/MD (n:2) Asymp
P11	0.60	0.04	0.26	2.2	0.41	0.06	5.9	13.7	c.1153C>T (p.Arg385Trp)	**c.1127T>C (p.Phe376Ser)**	BLD	C	3 years/ Asymp; I
P12[g]	0.56	0.05	0.25	4.0	0.36[e]	0.05[e]	3.0[e]	3.6[e]	**c.1220G>C (p.Gly407Ala)**	c.848T>C (p.Val283Ala)	4.0	M	2 years/ Asymp

Cases are ordered by decreasing C14:1 levels in DBS. Novel mutations are shown in bold

[a] VLCAD residual activity: % of intra-assay control; *BLD* below detection limit, *LF* lymphocytes, *NS* not studied

[b] Therapy: *L* low-LCT diet, *M* MCT supplement, *C* carnitine supplement (10–15 mg/kg/day)

[c] Clinical outcome: *Asymp* asymptomatic (normal anthropometric parameters; normal neurological and cardiological findings), *Hep* hepatopathy, *I* infections, *MD* metabolic decompensation, *Myo* myopathy, *HC* hypertrophic cardiomyopathy, *PST* paroxysmal supraventricular tachycardia

[d] *NR* normal range

[e] Plasma sample obtained >1 month

[f] DBS obtained at 12 days

[g] Siblings

Table 2 Clinical, biochemical, and molecular findings in suspected VLCADD cases identified by NBS with one or no mutations in *ACADVL*

	DBS (NBS) (48 h)				Plasma (confirmatory test)							
	C14:1 (μmol/L)	C14:1/C2	C14:1/C16	C14:1/C12:1	C14:1 (μmol/L) <1 month	C14:1/C2	C14:1/C16	C14:1/C12:1	Mutations in *ACADVL*[a]	VLCAD activity[b] (LF) (%)	Therapy	Age/clinical outcome[c]
NR[d]	<0.27–0.50	<0.015–0.030	<0.037–0.140	<7–7.3	<0.17	<0.023	<1.27	<5.69				
ID												
P13	2.20	0.123	0.40	7.33	0.50	0.080	2.94	5.0	**c.990_994delCAAGC (p.Lys331Cysfs*26) (no del)**	25	No	4 years/ Asymp
P14[e]	1.44	0.073	0.41	2.36	0.14	0.017	1.40	2.3	c.199A>T (p.Lys67Ter)	NS	No	12 months/ Asymp
P15	1.15	0.029	0.24	2.25	0.36	0.028	1.64	2.0	c.896_898delAGA (p.Lys299del)	57	No	21 months/ Asymp
P16	1.09	0.047	0.25	2.32	0.38	0.040	1.19	2.2	**c.1102_1103delCA (p.Gln368Valfs*26) (no del)**	20	No	4 years/ Asymp
P17	1.02	0.043	0.22	2.91	0.87	0.072	2.49	2.2	c.294_297delGACA (p.Gln98Hisfs*18)	18	No	3 years/ Asymp
P18[f]	0.93	0.031	0.15	2.74	0.15	0.016	1.50	3.0	c.896_898delAGA (p.Lys299del)	NS	No	12 months/ Asymp
P19[f]	0.87	0.033	0.21	2.72	0.13	0.014	1.18	3.3	c.896_898delAGA (p.Lys299del)	NS	No	12 months/ Asymp
P20	0.80	0.030	0.23	1.86	0.22	0.038	0.79	1.2	c.896_898delAGA (p.Lys299del)	33	No	2.5 years/ Asymp
P21	0.87	0.050	0.30	2.29	0.15	0.020	2.14	3.8	**c.515T>C (p.Leu172Pro) (no del)**	NS	No	4.5 years/ Asymp
P22	0.82	0.040	0.23	2.00	0.09	0.012	1.13	3.0	c.643T>C (p.Cys215Arg)	NS	No	17 months/ Asymp
P23	0.81	0.005	0.03	4.00	0.08	0.010	0.62	0.8	**c.1627T>C (p.Phe543Leu)**	34	No	2 years/ Asymp
P24	0.75	0.031	0.19	1.74	0.09	0.011	1.29	1.8	c.481G>A (p.Ala161Thr)	NS	No	14 months/ Asymp
P25	0.70	0.020	0.11	2.41	0.08	0.008	1.00	2.7	c.694G>A (p.Ala232Thr)	NS	No	14 months/ Asymp
P26	0.65	0.027	0.18	1.44	0.05	0.006	1.00	2.5	**c.1037C>T (p.Ala346Val)**	NS	No	20 months/ Asymp
P27	0.61	0.023	0.15	1.69	0.09	0.014	0.75	1.3	**c.1322G>C (p.Gly441Ala)**	NS	No	13 months/ Asymp
P28	0.46	0.02	0.14	1.39	0.20	0.010	0.87	1.3	c.272C>T (p.Pro91Leu)	NS	No	21 months/ Asymp

(continued)

Table 2 (continued)

NR[d]	DBS (NBS) (48 h)				Plasma (confirmatory test)				Mutations in ACADVL[a]	VLCAD activity[b] (LF) (%)	Therapy	Age/clinical outcome[c]
	C14:1 (µmol/L)	C14:1/ C2	C14:1/ C16	C14:1/ C12:1	C14:1 (µmol/L)	C14:1/ C2	C14:1/ C16	C14:1/ C12:1				
	0.27–0.50	0.015–0.030	0.037–0.140	7–7.3 (<1 month)	<0.17	<0.023	<1.27	<5.69				
P29	0.61	0.027	0.17	1.56	0.06	0.008	0.35	2.0	NS	57	No	14 months/ Asymp
P30	0.61	0.012	0.10	1.97	0.02	0.004	0.22	1.0	No mutations	NS	No	2.5 years/ Asymp
P31	0.59	0.026	0.14	1.28	0.03	0.004	0.43	1.5	No mutations	NS	No	18 months/ Asymp
P32	0.56	0.018	0.16	1.27	0.04	0.004	0.31	1.3	No mutations	NS	No	2 years/ Asymp
P33[e]	0.53	0.023	0.15	1.29	0.05	0.006	0.45	1.0	No mutations	NS	No	12 months/ Asymp
P34	0.52	0.023	0.14	1.33	0.02	0.003	0.40	1.0	No mutations	NS	No	14 months/ Asymp
P35	0.50	0.025	0.17	1.25	0.06	0.006	0.50	1.5	No mutations	NS	No	22 months/ Asymp
P36	0.44	0.024	0.11	1.22	0.05	0.008	0.83	1.3	No mutations	NS	No	18 months/ Asymp

Cases are ordered by decreasing C14:1 levels in DBS and genotype found. Novel mutations are in bold

[a] Mutations in *ACADVL*: *no del* no deletions

[b] VLCAD residual activity: % of intra-assay control; *LF* lymphocytes, *NS* not studied

[c] Clinical outcome: *Asymp* asymptomatic (normal anthropometric parameters; normal neurologic and cardiologic examination)

[d] *NR* normal range

[e] Fraternal twins

[f] Identical twins

shown), with at least one of the ratios in some cases (Tables 1 and 2). The predictive score for VLCADD was found informative in 31 out of 36 cases (condition "very likely" in P1–P10; P13, P14; P17; condition "likely" in P11; P15; P16; P18; P21; P22; and condition "possibly" in P12; P19; P20; P23–P26; P29; P31–P33; P35).

Confirmatory Testing

Classification

Cases were classified according to the results of the confirmatory tests. True-positive cases were those with abnormal plasma C14:1 levels and ratios, and with bi-allelic mutations coupled to deficient VLCAD activity in lymphocytes (<12% of intra-assay control: cases P1–P12). Individuals P11 and P12 displayed a mild increase in DBS C14:1 and they were later considered true-positive cases after completing the confirmatory testing. Disease carriers were considered P13–P29: those with only a mild increase in plasma C14:1 and of at least one ratio, the presence of only one single loss of function (LoF) mutation (P13–P20), or with one single probably missense mutation (P21–P28) and with intermediate residual activity (18–57%), and P29 (not genotyped) with just an intermediate activity of 57%. Those individuals with normal biochemical parameters and no mutations were classified as false positive cases (P30–P36).

Biochemical Confirmatory Analysis

Acylcarnitines were measured in plasma obtained between day 8 and 23 in all cases, except in cases P3 and P12 where it was obtained at 2 and 3 months of age, respectively. Sixteen cases (P1–P13, P15–P17) presented increased C14:1 levels (0.36–2.74 μmol/L; NV <0.17) with altered ratios in many of them. These parameters were normal in the remaining cases except for an isolated mild increase of C14:1 in P20 and P28 (Tables 1 and 2). Some overlapping in the plasma AC levels was observed between the true-positive cases and the disease carriers.

Significant differences in the C14:1 concentration were found between the 12 true-positive cases and the eight carriers of loss of function (LoF) mutations (P13–P20), both in DBS and plasma ($p < 0.01$). Similarly, the increases in the C14:1/C2, C14:1/C16, and C14:1/C12:1 ratios were also significant different in both groups ($p < 0.05$), with the increase in the C14:1/C16 ratio being the most significant parameter ($p < 0.005$) in both situations. The C14:1 concentrations were also significantly higher in both DBS and plasma ($p < 0.05$) among the carriers of LoF mutations (P13–P20) and the rest of heterozygotes (P21–P29), although in this case the ratios were not (Tables 1 and 2).

Secondary indicators of abnormal fatty acid oxidation, such as urine dicarboxylic and 3-hydroxydicarboxylic acids, were within normal limits in all the cases studied, except in individuals P2 and P14 who excreted medium-chain dicarboxylic acids (data not shown). The analysis of organic acids in urine proved to be uninformative.

Moreover, three asymptomatic mothers of heterozygous individuals (P13, P16, and P17) that carried the mutation found in their child, had a normal AC profile in DBS, ruling out maternal VLCADD (data not shown).

Molecular Analysis

A mutational analysis of *ACADVL* was performed on 35 individuals (33 unrelated families), of which 12 had bi-allelic variants (P1–P12), 16 only one pathogenic variant in the exonic region (P13–P28), and 7 carried no mutations (P30–P36, see Tables 1 and 2 for the genotypes). In total, 28 different variants were detected, including 12 that have not been previously reported: 8 potential missense changes and 4 severe LoF mutations. All the possible missense changes were predicted to be probably disease-causing mutations, affecting highly conserved residues in at least one algorithm used, and none of these were detected in control samples (Richards et al. 2015; Dopazo et al. 2016) (Table 3). All the individuals with bi-allelic changes carried at least one previously described or one LoF mutation, except P1.

Only one variant was detected in 16 individuals, 8 of whom carried a LoF mutation (Table 2), while 6 variants were new: 2 LoF (c.990_994delCAAGC; c.1102_1103delCA) and 4 probably missense mutations (c.515T>C; c.1037C>T; c.1322G>C; c.1627T>C). Genomic rearrangements were ruled out by CGH arrays in P13, P16, and P21. The most common mutations have already been described: c.848T>C (p.Val283Ala), six alleles; c.896_898delAGA (p.Lys299del), three alleles; [c.1097G>A; c.1844G>A] [p.Arg366His; p.Arg615Gln], three alleles; and c.643T>C (p.Cys215Arg), three alleles. Curiously, two mutations [p.Arg366His; p.Arg615Gln] were present in the same allele in two patients (P5, P10).

Lymphocyte Enzyme Activity

The VLCAD activity in lymphocytes from nine healthy adult subjects ranged from 0.95 to 6.85 nmol/min/mg protein, with a mean ($\pm$SD) value of 3.37 ($\pm$1.99) nmol/min/mg protein. Enzyme activity of 0.015 and 0.135 nmol/min/mg protein (0.6 and 5.8% of the intra-assay control) was determined in two confirmed adult myopathic VLCAD-deficient patients to validate the method. The enzyme activity in lymphocytes was clearly deficient in 11 individuals with abnormal NBS results and 2 bi-allelic mutations, ranging from undetectable

Table 3 In silico prediction of novel missense variations in *ACADVL*

| Nucleotide variation | Protein effect | Alamut® Visual | | | | | | | |
		SIFT	Mutation Taster	Poliphen-2	ExAC	Splicing prediction	Provean	Mutation assessor	CSVS
c.515T>C	p.Leu172Pro	Tolerated (score: 0.1)	Disease causing	Benign 0.131	0	No	Deleterious	Low	0
c.761G>A	p.Gly254Asp	Deleterious (score: 0)	Disease causing	Probably damaging 0.992	0	No	Deleterious	Low	0
c.1037C>T	p.Ala346Val	Deleterious (score: 0)	Disease causing	Probably damaging 0.964	0	No	Deleterious	Medium	0
c.1127T>C	p.Phe376Ser	Deleterious (score: 0.01)	Disease causing	Possibly damaging 0.639	0.000082	No	Deleterious	High	0
c.1174G>C	p.Val392Leu	Tolerated (score: 0.09)	Disease causing	Possibly damaging 0.680	0	No	Neutral	Low	0
c.1220G>C	p.Gly407Ala	Deleterious (score: 0)	Disease causing	Probably damaging 0.941	0	No	Deleterious	Medium	0
c.1322G>C	p.Gly441Ala	Deleterious (score: 0)	Disease causing	Possibly damaging 0.778	0	No	Deleterious	High	0
c.1627T>C	p.Phe543Leu	Deleterious (score: 0)	Disease causing	Benign 0.418	0	No	Deleterious	Medium	0

Alamut® *Visual* http://www.interactive-biosoftware.com/doc/alamut-visual (GRCh38, RS758928307)
Splicing prediction SpliceSiteFinder-like, MaxEntScan, NNSPLICE, GeneSplicer, Human Splicing Finder (HSF)
Provean http://provean.jcvi.org/index.php
Mutation assessor http://mutationassessor.org/r3/
CSVS http://csvs.babelomics.org/

to 11.8% of the simultaneous control (Table 1). There was residual activity in five cases with only one LoF mutation in *ACADVL* (P13, P15, P16, P17, and P20), ranging from 18 to 57% of the intra-assay control (Table 2). The enzyme activity was also reduced in P23 (34%), an individual carrying one novel missense variant, and in P29 (57%) that has not yet been genotyped. The enzyme activity in five parents carrying one mutation in *ACADVL* ranged from 0.43 to 1.31 nmol/min/mg protein (34.7–40% of the intra-assay control).

Clinical and Biochemical Outcome

Clinical questionnaires were completed for 36 cases from 33 families. The parents of most individuals were of Spanish origin (18 families), there were 4 from Morocco, 2 from Romania, 2 from China, 1 from Peru, 1 from Venezuela, and 6 mixed couples (Spain-Hispanic). Consanguinity was only recognized in the family of P1 and no incidents of interest were reported in any of the pregnancies. There were three twin pregnancies (two identical and one fraternal), and both children of two of these pregnancies (P14 and P33; P18 and P19) and only one from the third (P23) were investigated. One of these pregnancies was a preterm labor, and in the whole cohort five cesarean deliveries were documented. All cases were asymptomatic when referred to clinical units, except four cases that were admitted to hospital in the neonatal period (between 1 and 15 days) due to dehydration and weight loss (P2), paroxysmal supraventricular tachycardia (P5), jaundice (P16), or prematurity (P23, twin pregnancy), all without metabolic decompensation. Seven true-positive individuals were admitted to hospital due to different infections between 3 months and 4 years of age, usually gastroenteritis, gingival stomatitis or pneumonia, and these symptoms were accompanied by metabolic decompensation in four of these cases (P1, P3, P7 and P10). These individuals presented elevated creatine kinase (CK: 515–4,000 U/L), elevated transaminases, hypoglycemia, and/or metabolic acidosis. In addition, P3 was admitted several times for emergency treatment due to severe metabolic decompensation, usually presenting increased CK (515–1,296 U/L, N 26–308) even when stable.

The decision whether or not to treat the children, and what is the optimal treatment for each patient, is difficult as there are currently no evidence-based guidelines available. For each individual patient clinical decision making was based on the consensus recommendations of European experts (Spiekerkoetter et al. 2009). Asymptomatic cases with normal values of glucose, CK and liver enzymes were fed with a 50:50 mixture of breast milk (or infant formula) mixed with a special medium-chain triglyceride (MCT)-enriched infant formula, which was prescribed according to age in order to avoid fasting. A specific appropriate sick day regime was also provided. After confirmatory studies,

dietary intervention was recommended in those cases with two mutations and low residual activity. A fat modified diet (LCT ≤10% of total caloric value and MCT 20% of total caloric value) and carnitine (15–50 mg/kg/day) were administered to 6 of the 12 children. Only MCT supplementation was provided to 3 of the 12, LCT restriction and MCT supplementation in 1, LCT restriction and carnitine in 1, and only carnitine supplementation in another (Table 1). The follow-up period of the individuals varied between 12 months and 5.5 years. All the evaluated individuals except one (P3) are in good condition, with normal growth and anthropometric parameters (weight, height and head circumference), normal psychomotor development and neurologic examination, normal cardiologic examination with normal ECG record and normal routine biochemical parameters without hepatic or muscle impairment. To date, P3 is the only clinically affected individual despite adhering to a regulated diet, with several decompensated parameters, hypertrophic cardiomyopathy, hepatopathy, myopathy, and hypotonia at 3 years of age.

The plasma AC levels were monitored periodically in ten true-positive cases and six carriers of LoF mutations. Under treatment, plasma C14:1 levels remained high (1.01–3.4 µmol/L) in cases P1, P2, P5, and P7, all with very low residual activity (<5%), who were in good clinical condition and complied well with their diet. By contrast, in six cases the plasma AC levels were only slightly higher than the controls (0.17–0.50 µmol/L): P4, P6, P8, P9, P10, and P12. Carriers that did not receive dietary interventions always had C14:1 levels in the control range (<0.17 µmol/L), except P13 who had levels slightly above those of the controls (0.21–0.50 µmol/L).

Discussion

Although the detection of VLCADD is not mandatory in Spanish expanded NBS programs, it is included in some regions because the early detection of this disease may improve the outcome if prophylactic measures are rapidly put in place. The true incidence of VLCADD in Spain is not known and in fact, between 1989 and 2010 very few cases were diagnosed based on clinical evidence: five patients in Madrid (three with severe early onset and two with adolescent myopathic presentation) (Merinero et al. 1996); and at least three cases in Barcelona (Osorio et al. 2003). In some Spanish regions, no positive cases were identified between 2000 and 2013 in more than 800,000 newborns screened in the expanded NBS programs (approximately 46% of all annual births (Rocha et al. 2014)). Hence, the high number of cases with suspected VLCADD that were detected here over a short period (between April 2011 and December 2015) was quite striking. In order to better understand how this increased incidence arose, we first set out to unambiguously distinguish the true-positive cases that need nutritional intervention and clinical monitoring from those individuals that are carriers of the disease, or even false-positive cases. To achieve this we revised the results of the NBS and of the diagnostic evaluation (plasma AC profiles, molecular findings, lymphocyte enzyme activity), as well as the clinical outcome and treatment data of 36 cases detected by NBS in the last 4 years.

Initially, the combination of plasma AC profile and mutational analysis was used to confirm the diagnosis of VLCADD. However, most of the cases presented only one exonic mutation, although other nucleotide changes in the proximal or distal promoter or in deep intronic sequences could not be ruled out because routine genetic analysis only involves the sequencing of coding exonic regions. Besides, the finding of novel mutations with uncertain clinical significance in some cases makes it more complicated to achieve a true diagnosis of VLCADD, as occurred elsewhere (Schiff et al. 2013).

The determination of enzyme activity in lymphocytes was added to the diagnostic algorithm in order to provide accurate information for clinicians. All the cases with two bi-allelic mutations had low residual activity (<12%), even the cases bearing the mild p.Val283Ala mutation (Andresen et al. 1999). By contrast, those cases with only one nucleotide change presented intermediate residual activity that ranged from 18 to 57%, suggesting that they were indeed carriers of the disease. In our hands, the determination of enzyme activity in lymphocytes proved useful as a rapid confirmatory test to definitively classify the cases into true-positive cases or carriers. There is a lack of correlation between VLCAD enzyme activity in lymphocytes and AC levels in DBS and plasma samples in our confirmed patients. Similar inconsistencies between the biochemical data, genetic results, enzyme studies, and/or presence of clinical symptoms have already been described; therefore, the need to combine different confirmatory tests. The enzyme activity also does not allow carriers to be discriminated from healthy controls, as occurs elsewhere (ter Veld et al. 2009).

The fact that with nutritional therapy 11 true-positive patients remain free of symptoms after a mean follow-up of 30 months, and only one is symptomatic, highlights the importance of early diagnosis through NBS and prompt nutritional intervention. Nevertheless, early intervention does not prevent asymptomatic cases from being at risk of presenting symptoms in the future and hence, such cases will require close clinical monitoring, especially in situations of energy demand (fasting, prolonged exercise, illness, adolescence, etc.). In this cohort the disease carriers did not present any symptoms, despite a mild increase in plasma C14:1 during the follow-up period. Thus, it would seem that they are not at risk of developing clinical complications in the future and therefore, a clinical and biochemical follow-up may not be necessary.

In our experience the R4S post-analytical tool has allowed to discriminate most true-positive cases as very likely/likely (P1–P11) except P12 and there were no false negative cases. The evaluation of five clearly false positive cases (P27, P28, P30, P34, and P36) could have been avoided. So, the R4S post-analytical tool is able to provide reliable advice on the interpretation of NBS results.

Although the increase in the number of cases with suspected VLCADD may be at least partially related to the different cut-offs used in the regional NBS centers, it seems that this disease is more common in Spain than previously thought. Based on this experience, we suggest that cases with abnormal plasma C14:1 (>1 μmol/L) and with higher ratios of C14:1/C2, C14:1/C16 and/or C14:1/C12:1 will need early dietary treatment pending the outcome of the enzymatic/molecular analysis. We recommend that enzyme analysis should be performed in all newborns with mild plasma C14:1 levels ranging from 0.36 to 1 μmol/L in order to definitively classify them as true-positive cases or disease carriers, and to decide which will require treatment, as well as clinical and biochemical monitoring. Moreover, in those children with normal plasma results in the first 6 months of life, no further biochemical studies are needed.

Conclusions

This is the first time that data has been compiled on suspected VLCADD cases identified through NBS programs in Spain. True-positive cases were defined as those with increased C14:1 and ratios, two pathogenic mutations and deficient VLCAD activity in lymphocytes. All these individuals are receiving a nutritional intervention and to date, all but one remain asymptomatic. Children with normal or only a mild increase in plasma C14:1, the presence of only one single mutation and intermediate residual activity don't seem to be at risk of developing clinical complications in the future and a close follow-up is not necessary. Enzyme determination is essential in many cases to interpret the genetic findings and to decide which cases require treatment, as well as close clinical and biochemical monitoring. Using biochemical, enzymatic, and comprehensive gene analysis, a biochemical genetic service could rapidly evaluate potential patients.

Acknowledgments The authors would like to thank the families involved in this study for giving their consent. This work was funded by a grant from the Fundación Isabel Gemio. The authors confirm independence from the sponsors; the content of the article has not been influenced by the sponsors.

A Concise One Sentence Take-Home Message

The combined evaluation of the acylcarnitine profiles, genetic results, and residual enzyme activities have proven useful to definitively classify individuals with suspected VLCAD deficiency into true-positive cases and carriers, and to decide which cases need treatment, as well as close clinical and biochemical monitoring.

Compliance with Ethics Guidelines

Conflict of Interests

None of the authors have any conflict of interests to declare.

Informed Consent

All procedures followed were in accordance with the ethical standards of the responsible committee on human experimentation and with the Helsinki Declaration of 1975, as revised in 2000 (5). This project was approved by the Universidad Autónoma Madrid Ethics Committee (reference number CEI 74-1349).

Details of the Contributions of Individuals Authors

All authors approved the final manuscript as submitted.

BM: conception and design, drafting, and coordination of the manuscript.

PA: enzyme activity determinations, statistical analysis, and writing the first draft.

EMH: treating metabolic specialist of patients, drafting of the manuscript.

AM: treating metabolic specialist of patients.

MTGS: treating metabolic specialist of patients.

PQF: treating metabolic specialist of patients.

CPG: treating metabolic specialist of patients.

ED: analysis and interpretation of newborn screening data from Madrid.

RY: analysis and interpretation of newborn screening data from Western Andalucia.

JME: analysis and interpretation of newborn screening data from Murcia.

ABQ: treating metabolic specialist of patients.

JBA: treating metabolic specialist of patients.

MLFR: analysis and interpretation of newborn screening data from Madrid.

BB: analysis of newborn screening data from Madrid.

IFL: acylcarnitines and organic acids analysis.

FL: molecular genetic analysis.

MU: critical review of the manuscript for important intellectual content.

PRS: biochemical and enzyme data analysis.

BP: molecular genetic data interpretation, drafting of the manuscript.

CPC: biochemical data interpretation, drafting of the manuscript.

References

Andresen BS, Olpin S, Poorthuis BJ, Scholte HR et al (1999) Clear correlation of genotype with disease phenotype in very-long-chain acyl-CoA dehydrogenase deficiency. Am J Hum Genet 64: 479–494

Arnold GL, Van Hove J, Freedenberg D, Strauss A et al (2009) A Delphi clinical practice protocol for the management of very long chain acyl-CoA dehydrogenase deficiency. Mol Genet Metab 96:85–90

Boneh A, Andresen BS, Gregersen N, Ibrahim M et al (2006) VLCAD deficiency: pitfalls in newborn screening and confirmation of diagnosis by mutation analysis. Mol Genet Metab 88: 166–170

Browning MF, Larson C, Strauss A, Marsden DL (2005) Normal acylcarnitine levels during confirmation of abnormal newborn screening in long-chain fatty acid oxidation defects. J Inherit Metab Dis 28:545–550

Coughlin CR 2nd, Ficicioglu C (2010) Genotype-phenotype correlations: sudden death in an infant with very-long-chain acyl-CoA dehydrogenase deficiency. J Inherit Metab Dis 33(Suppl 3): S129–S131

Dopazo J, Amadoz A, Bleda M, Garcia-Alonso L et al (2016) 267 Spanish exomes reveal population-specific differences in disease-related genetic variation. Mol Biol Evol 33:1205–1218

Ferrer I, Ruiz-Sala P, Vicente Y, Merinero B et al (2007) Separation and identification of plasma short-chain acylcarnitine isomers by HPLC/MS/MS for the differential diagnosis of fatty acid oxidation defects and organic acidemias. J Chromatogr B 860: 121–126

Hall PL, Marquardt G, McHugh DM, Currier RJ et al (2014) Postanalytical tools improve performance of newborn screening by tandem mass spectrometry. Genet Med 16:889–895

Merinero B, Perez-Cerda C, Garcia MJ, Gangoiti J et al (1996) Mitochondrial very long-chain acyl-CoA dehydrogenase deficiency with a mild clinical course. J Inherit Metab Dis 19: 173–176

Merinero B, Pascual Pascual SI, Perez-Cerda C, Gangoiti J et al (1999) Adolescent myopathic presentation in two sisters with very long-chain acyl-CoA dehydrogenase deficiency. J Inherit Metab Dis 22:802–810

Merritt JL 2nd, Vedal S, Abdenur JE, Au SM et al (2014) Infants suspected to have very-long chain acyl-CoA dehydrogenase deficiency from newborn screening. Mol Genet Metab 111: 484–492

Osorio JH, Lluch M, Ribes A (2003) Analysis of organic acids after incubation with (16-2H3)palmitic acid in fibroblasts from patients with mitochondrial beta-oxidation defects. J Inherit Metab Dis 26:795–803

Pena LD, van Calcar SC, Hansen J, Edick MJ et al (2016) Outcomes and genotype-phenotype correlations in 52 individuals with

VLCAD deficiency diagnosed by NBS and enrolled in the IBEM-IS database. Mol Genet Metab 118:272–281

Richards S, Aziz N, Bale S, Bick D et al (2015) Standards and guidelines for the interpretation of sequence variants: a joint consensus recommendation of the American College of Medical Genetics and Genomics and the Association for Molecular Pathology. Genet Med 17:405–424

Rocha H, Castineiras D, Delgado C, Egea J et al (2014) Birth prevalence of fatty acid beta-oxidation disorders in Iberia. JIMD Rep 16:89–94

Schiff M, Mohsen AW, Karunanidhi A, McCracken E et al (2013) Molecular and cellular pathology of very-long-chain acyl-CoA dehydrogenase deficiency. Mol Genet Metab 109:21–27

Spiekerkoetter U, Lindner M, Santer R, Grotzke M et al (2009) Treatment recommendations in long-chain fatty acid oxidation defects: consensus from a workshop. J Inherit Metab Dis 32:498–505

Spiekerkoetter U, Haussmann U, Mueller M, ter Veld F et al (2010) Tandem mass spectrometry screening for very long-chain acyl-CoA dehydrogenase deficiency: the value of second-tier enzyme testing. J Pediatr 157:668–673

Tajima G, Sakura N, Yofune H, Nishimura Y et al (2005) Enzymatic diagnosis of medium-chain acyl-CoA dehydrogenase deficiency by detecting 2-octenoyl-CoA production using high-performance liquid chromatography: a practical confirmatory test for tandem mass spectrometry newborn screening in Japan. J Chromatogr B 823:122–130

ter Veld F, Mueller M, Kramer S, Haussmann U et al (2009) A novel tandem mass spectrometry method for rapid confirmation of medium- and very long-chain acyl-CoA dehydrogenase deficiency in newborns. PLoS One 4:e6449

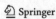

JIMD Reports
DOI 10.1007/8904_2017_47

RESEARCH REPORT

Social Functioning and Behaviour in Mucopolysaccharidosis IH [Hurlers Syndrome]

Annukka Lehtonen · Stewart Rust · Simon Jones ·
Richard Brown · Dougal Hare

Received: 17 November 2016 / Revised: 29 June 2017 / Accepted: 03 July 2017 / Published online: 29 July 2017
© Society for the Study of Inborn Errors of Metabolism (SSIEM) 2017

Abstract *Background*: Mucopolysaccharidosis type IH (MPS-IH) [Hurlers Syndrome] is a developmental genetic disorder characterised by severe physical symptoms and cognitive decline. This study aimed to investigate the behavioural phenotype of MPS-IH treated by haematopoietic cell transplantation, focusing on social functioning and sleep. Parental stress was also measured.

Methods: Participants were 22 children with MPS-IH (mean age 9 years 1 month), of whom 10 were male (45%). Parents completed the Social Responsiveness Scale (SRS), Child Behaviour Checklist (CBCL), Children's Sleep Habit Questionnaire and Parent Stress Index, Short Form (PSI-SF).

Results: Twenty-three per cent of children with MPS-IH scored in the severe range of the SRS, suggesting significant difficulties in social functioning. Children with MPS-IH were more than 30 times more likely to receive scores in the severe range than typically developing children. Thirty-six per cent scored in the mild-to-moderate range, suggesting milder, but marked, difficulties in social interaction. Although children with MPS-IH did not show significantly higher rates of internalising, externalising or total behaviour problems than the normative sample, they received scores that were significantly higher on social, thought and attention problems and rule-breaking behaviour, and all the competence areas of the CBCL. Parents of children with MPS-IH did not score significantly higher on parental stress than parents in a normative sample.

Conclusions: Parents of children with MPS-IH rate their children as having problems with social functioning and various areas of competence more frequently than previously thought, with implications for clinical support.

Communicated by: Olaf Bodamer, MD PhD

A. Lehtonen · R. Brown
Division of Psychology and Mental Health, School of Health Sciences, Faculty of Biology, Medicine and Health, University of Manchester, Manchester, UK

S. Rust
Paediatric Psychosocial Department, Royal Manchester Children's Hospital, Manchester, UK

S. Jones
Willink Unit, Manchester Centre for Genomic Medicine, St Mary's Hospital, Central Manchester University Hospitals NHS Foundation Trust (CMFT), University of Manchester, Manchester, UK

D. Hare (✉)
Wales Autism Research Centre, School of Psychology, Cardiff University, Cardiff, UK
e-mail: hared@cardiff.ac.uk

Introduction

Mucopolysaccharidosis type I (MPS-I) is an autosomal recessive genetic disorder with a frequency of 1.07/100,000 in England and Wales (Moore et al. 2008). The most severe subtype, Hurler syndrome (MPS-IH), is characterised by early onset of symptoms and central nervous system (CNS) involvement. MPS-I is chronic and progressive, affecting multiple bodily systems (D'Aco et al. 2012) with symptom onset in infancy and early cognitive decline due to CNS damage. MPS-I is caused by deficient alpha-L iduronidase enzyme and consequent inability to metabolise glycosaminoglycans (GAGs), which accumulate causing tissue dysfunction.

Children with MPS-IH are currently treated with haematopoietic stem cell transplantation (HCT), which has reduced morbidity and mortality but not eliminated all disease burden. Post-HCT enzyme activity in white cells is similar to that of healthy individuals and the accumulated GAGs disappear or decrease. HCT halts cognitive decline; however, general learning problems persist with post-HCT cognitive scores tending to be 1 SD lower than population mean (Eisengart et al. 2013; Aldenhoven et al. 2015; Shapiro et al. 2015).

Few studies have investigated behaviour in children with MPS-IH. Krivit et al. (1995) suggested that children with MPS-IH only display behaviour problems later in their development. Bax and Colville (1995) reported sleep problems, fearfulness and difficulty to settle, and Bjoraker et al. (2006) noted that children with MPS-IH had deficits in various areas of adaptive functioning, making progress at a slower rate than typically developing children. The latter may be partly due to residual post-treatment hearing and movement difficulties.

Other aspects of the MPS-IH behavioural phenotype that have been examined include social functioning, with Bjoraker et al. (2006) reporting impairments compared to normative data and Pitt et al. (2009) reporting that children with MPS-IH participate in social activities less than typically developing children. Sleep problems have also been identified as a problem in MPS-I disorders (1995), although not specifically in MPS-IH. Given the significant effect that a child's sleeping problems can have on family functioning (Quine 1991, 1992; Wiggs and Stores 2001), further investigation is important. Parental stress is another factor potentially influencing quality of life for children with MPS-IH and their families, as parents of children with chronic illnesses have been shown to report significantly higher stress levels than parents of healthy children (Cousino and Hazen 2013). Furthermore, parental stress is associated with parental depression (Driscoll et al. 2010) and child behaviour problems (Colletti et al. 2008).

The aim of this study was to investigate the behavioural phenotype of children with MPS-IH compared to published norms and children with intellectual disability, with a specific focus on social functioning and sleep. Parental stress was also examined.

Method

Recruitment

MPS-IH Group

The majority of the children with MPS-IH diagnosis were recruited from the Northwest of England. The parents/guardians of eligible children were sent a study pack including an introductory letter, information sheet, consent form, parental questionnaires and a freepost envelope. If the parents/guardians had not responded within 4 weeks, they were telephoned to check they had received the questionnaire pack and to offer help in completing the questionnaires. Participants were also recruited through the UK MPS Society. Participants were excluded if they were outside the 2.5- to 16-year age range or if the parents did not have sufficient English to complete the questionnaires without an interpreter.

Comparison Group

A comparison group of children with mixed intellectual disabilities was recruited via the Facebook pages of the charities Cerebra and MENCAP and via 69 schools for children with special needs in England, selected through EduBase. Exclusion criteria were age ≤2.5 years or ≥16 years and/or an autistic spectrum disorder (ASD) diagnosis or genetic disorder associated with ASD (e.g. fragile X syndrome).

Measures

Social Responsiveness Scale, 2nd edition (SRS-2) (Constantino 2012): The 65-item standardised questionnaire identifying social impairment typical in ASD, over five subscales (*Social Awareness, Social Cognition, Social Communication, Social Motivation, Restricted Interests and Repetitive Behaviour*). Versions for both the preschoolers (2.5- to 4.5-year olds) and school-age children (4- to 18-year olds) were used. Internal consistency is good ($\alpha = 0.92–0.95$) and clinical cut-offs for severe (≥ 75) and mild-to-moderate (61–74) levels of ASD symptomatology are provided. The rates of typically developing children receiving scores above the clinical cut-off (for PDD-NOS, 101.5) are 1.4% for boys and 0.3% for girls (Constantino and Todd 2003).

Child Behaviour Checklist (CBCL; Achenbach and Rescorla 2001): The 100-item version for ages 1.5–5 years and the 120-item version for ages 6–18 years were used to generate scores for internalising and externalising problems, total problems score and various syndrome scores. The version for 6- to 18-year olds also included competence scales, equivalent to measures of adaptive behaviour described in literature. Internal consistency for the CBCL ranged from 0.63 to 0.97.

Children's Sleep Habits Rating Scale: A 36-item measure adapted from the Children's Sleep Habits Questionnaire (Owens et al. 2000) by Mahon et al. (2014) to assess whether a range of sleep problems occur "usually" (5–7 nights a week), "sometimes" (2–4 times a week) or rarely (0–1 time a week).

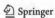

Parenting Stress Index, short form (PSI-SF; Abidin 1995): A 36-item scale to identify characteristics of family functioning and parenting that may hinder normal development and functioning. The PSI-SF provides three sub-scores (*parental distress, parent-child dysfunctional interaction* and *difficult child*) and a total score. It is standardised for children aged up to 12-year olds.

In addition, the parents of 16 children gave consent to access routinely collected IQ scores variously derived from the *Wechsler Intelligence Scale for Children, 4th Edition* (WISC-IV), Wechsler Preschool and Primary Scale of Intelligence, 3rd Edition (WPPSI-III) and *The Bayley Scales for Infant and Toddler Development, 3rd Edition.*

Statistical Analyses

Data were analysed in SPSS version 22 with alpha $= p < 0.05$. Normality of distributions was assessed using Kolmogorov–Smirnov tests. Differences between participants/non-participants were investigated by t-tests and χ^2 tests. Differences between MPS-IH group and norms on the outcome measures were explored by one-sample t-tests and Wilcoxon Signed Rank Tests. Odds ratios were computed to examine the rates of clinical scores on the SRS in the MPS-IH sample compared to typically developing children. Regression analysis was used to investigate the relationship between IQ and SRS total scores to check that the former was not a confounding variable. For the CBCL, raw scores were used for normative comparisons, as T scores are truncated at 50 and therefore not necessarily sensitive for variation at the low end of syndrome T scores or high end of competence T scores.

Results

Thirty-five children were identified as eligible for the study from the clinical database; of these, twenty-one were enrolled into the study (60%), with two more children with MPS-IH enrolled through the MPS Society. Fifteen families expressed interest in participating in the control arm of the study but as only nine completed the questionnaires, these data were not used and the scores of the children with MPS-IH were compared to available norms.

Since the demographic information (age and gender) was available for all the eligible children in the clinical database, it was possible to analyse whether the children whose parents were enrolled into the study ("participants") were significantly different on these measures than the children whose parents were not enrolled into the study ("non-participants"). This analysis was not possible for the MPS Society recruits as the demographics of potential participants were not available. Table 1 presents the demographic information for

Table 1 Demographic details of the responders and non-responders of the patient sample

	Responders $N = 21$	Non-responders $N = 14$
Male/female	9/12	9/5
Mean age (SD)	9 years 7 months (4 years 2 months)	9 years 7 months (3 years 11 months)

Table 2 SRS and IQ scores

	Mean (SD)
SRS total T score	63.77 (14.72)
SRS total raw score (school-age)	67.69 (42.13)
SRS total raw score (preschool age)	75.67 (32.40)
SRS subscales	
Awareness	60.95 (12.45)
Cognition	65.18 (14.94)
Communication	61.23 (14.44)
Motivation	59.05 (14.28)
Restricted interests and repetitive behaviour (RRB)	66.09 (14.83)
IQ score	76.13 (22.98)

the participants and non-participants of the children on the clinical database. These groups did not significantly differ in terms of age ($t(33) = 0.042$, $p = 0.96$, CI [-2.81, 2.93]) or gender (χ^2 (1, $N = 35$) $= 1.54$, $p = 0.214$) and the mean age of the whole sample was 9 years 1 month (SD $= 4$ years 6 months); 45% were male (10/22).

The SRS scores of 23% (5/22) of the MPS-IH children were in the severe range of autism, 36% (8/22) in the mild-to-moderate range and 41% (9/22) in the normal range (Table 2). Mean total raw score for the school-age children with MPS-IH ($M = 67.7$, $SD = 42.1$) was significantly higher than the normative mean score ($M = 24.6$, $t(15) = 4.09$, $p = 0.001$, 95% CI [20.6, 65.5]). The mean total raw score for the preschool age children ($M = 75.7$, $SD = 32.4$) was not significantly different to the reported mean ($M = 42.5$), although there was a near-significant trend ($t(5) = 2.51$, $p = 0.054$, 95% CI [-0.84, 67.17]). Of the five subscales of the SRS, the social cognition subscale had the highest percentage of children scoring in the severe range.

A multiple regression analysis was conducted with age and IQ as independent variables and SRS total as a dependent variable. As the IQ scores were provided by different instruments, the total scores were standardised across measures and these scores were used in the regression analysis. The regression analysis indicated no significant effects of age or IQ on the SRS scores.

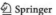

Odds ratios indicated that, compared to the rate for boys in Constantino and Todd (2003), children with MPS-IH were >31 times more likely to receive scores in the clinical range (OR = 31.64, 95% CI [5.66–176.61]).

Mean T scores and mean raw scores for the CBCL are shown in Table 3. Of the MPS-IH children, 24% (5/21) received scores in the clinical range for internalising problems, 19% (4/21) for externalising problems and 29% (6/21) for total problems.

The scores of the school-age children were compared to published norms. The internalising, externalising and total problem scores were normally distributed, while the sub-scores relating to *anxious/depressed, withdrawn/depressed, rule-breaking* and *aggression* were not. These data were therefore analysed using one-sample Wilcoxon Signed Rank Tests.

School-age children with MPS-IH did not significantly differ from the normative sample in their internalisation, externalisation or total problem scores, but had significantly more social problems (t(14) = 2.206, p = 0.045, 95% CI

[0.05, 3.88]), thought problems (t(14) = 3.152, p = 0.007, 95% CI [0.99, 5.18]), attention problems (t(14) = 2.598, p = 0.021, 95% CI [0.62, 6.64]) and demonstrated significantly more rule-breaking behaviour (Z = 24, p = 0.038) than the normative sample.

Preschool children with MPS-IH had significantly more attention problems (t(5) = 2.74, p = 0.041, 95% CI [0.26, 8.07]) and internalisation problems (t(5) = 2.86, p = 0.035, 95% CI [1.16, 21.84]) than the normative sample, but as there were N = 6 preschool-aged children, these findings should be regarded as illustrative only.

The CBCL competency scores were only available in the school-age CBCL and due to missing data, were only computable for 13 children, of whom 9 (69%) received scores in the clinical range in total competence, 31% (4/13) received scores in the clinical range for activities, 8% (1/14) for social competence and 31% (4/13) for school competence.

Comparisons to published norms indicated that children with MPS-IH received significantly lower scores on activities (t(12) = −5.00, p < 0.001, 95% CI [−5.49, −2.16]), social

Table 3 CBCL scores

School-age children	Mean T score (SD)	Mean raw score (SD)	Normative score	Significance	Effect size d
Anxious/depressed	54.40 (7.83)	2.67 (3.98)	3.00	n.s.	
Withdrawn/depressed	54.33 (7.70)	1.60 (2.80)	1.65	n.s.	
Somatic complaints	56.67 (7.37)	2.20 (2.51)	1.20	n.s.	
Social problems	58.20 (8.04)	4.07 (3.45)	2.10	*	0.57
Thought problems	61.60 (9.91)	4.73 (3.79)	1.65	*	0.81
Attention problems	62.07 (12.17)	7.13 (5.44)	3.50	*	0.67
Rule-breaking behaviour	53.27 (4.23)	1.53 (1.42)	2.05	*	
Aggressive behaviour	54.33 (6.75)	4.27 (5.12)	4.60	n.s.	
Internalising	49.67 (12.28)	6.47 (8.54)	50.15	n.s.	
Externalising	48.60 (10.64)	5.80 (6.22)	50.10	n.s.	
Total problems	53.93 (11.49)	32.27 (24.34)	49.80	n.s.	
Competence scales					
Activities	35.85 (7.84)	7.27 (2.76)	11.1	*	1.39
Social	40.31 (8.67)	6.23 (2.35)	8.75	*	1.07
School	34.54 (6.68)	3.10 (0.98)	5.05	*	2.00
Total competence	32.92 (8.31)	16.60 (4.13)	50.00	*	2.05
Preschool children					
Emotionally reactive	60.50 (7.77)	5.17 (2.86)	2.4	n.s.	
Anxious/depressed	54.50 (4.97)	3.00 (2.19)	2.9	n.s.	
Somatic complaints	63.50 (11.08)	5.17 (4.07)	1.8	n.s.	
Withdrawn	63.67 (9.09)	4.17 (2.71)	1.5	n.s.	
Sleep problems	58.67 (13.95)	3.67 (4.97)	2.8	n.s.	
Attention problems	70.50 (8.96)	6.67 (3.72)	2.5	*	1.12
Aggressive behaviour	59.00 (8.63)	14.50 (9.03)	10.4	n.s.	
Internalising	61.50 (9.85)	17.50 (9.48)	50.0	*	1.17
Externalising	59.33 (13.87)	21.17 (12.14)	50.0	n.s.	
Total problems	61.17 (12.31)	57.50 (28.72)	50.1	n.s.	

Table 4 Sleep and PSI-SF scores

Children's Sleep Habits Rating Scale	Mean (SD)
Sleep resistance	9.52 (3.76)
Sleep delay	1.71 (0.78)
Sleep onset delay	
Sleep anxiety	5.00 (2.07)
Sleep duration	5.62 (1.78)
Sleep waking	5.38 (1.91)
Night behaviours	2.43 (0.75)
Parasomnias	8.24 (2.05)
Breathing	5.10 (1.58)
Sleepiness	12.00 (2.86)
Total	54.85 (11.57)
PSI total stress	82.3 (25.9)
Parental distress	30.5 (10.6)
Dysfunctional interaction	22.9 (7.4)
Difficult child	29.2 (10.6)

skills ($t(12) = -3.86$, $p = 0.002$, 95% CI [3.94, −1.10]), school ($t(12) = -7.202$, $p < 0.001$, 95% CI [−2.54, −1.36]) and total competence ($t(12) = -7.41$, $p < 0.001$, 95% CI [−22.10, −12.05]).

Analysis of sleep data was based on a sample of 21, with parents reporting 57% (12/21) of their children to have sleep problems, with a median age of onset of 0 years (i.e. from birth; range = 0–13 years). Sleep problems included difficulties falling asleep, not getting tired and restless sleep. Five children had been prescribed melatonin (Table 4).

Fifty per cent of the children with MPS-IH usually fell asleep within 20 min, while 20% rarely or never did. Twenty per cent of the children with MPS-IH woke up more than once a night, 55% rarely or never. Only 15% of the children usually displayed disruptive behaviour; no children displayed dangerous behaviour. Sleep disordered breathing was shown by 5–6 children (loud snoring, snorting and gasping).

Since the PSI-SF is only normed for children aged 12 years and younger, data from 19 families are reported (Table 4), with five parents (26%) scoring in the clinically elevated range for the total score (>90; Abidin 1995). The mean total raw score of the parents of children with MPS-IH was not significantly higher than that of the normative sample ($M = 71.0$), however.

Discussion

The aim of this study was to investigate behaviour, particularly social functioning and sleep, and parental stress in children with MPS-IH. This is the first investigation of these factors in MPS-IH. The current data indicated that 23% of children with MPS-IH had clinically significant difficulties in social functioning likely to cause severe interference with everyday social interactions, with another 36% having similar but less pronounced difficulties. Moreover, the mean SRS score of the school-age MPS-IH group was significantly higher than that reported for typically developing children, and children with MPS-IH were 30 times more likely to receive scores in the severe clinical range than typically developing children. The difference between preschool-age children with MPS-IH and typically developing children did not reach significance, most likely due to the small sample size. These findings indicate that difficulties in social functioning and behaviours are more common in MPS-IH than previously thought.

In contrast, school-age children with MPS-IH showed no more internalising, externalising or general problem behaviour than their typically developing peers. Analysis of syndrome scores suggested that children with MPS-IH had significantly more social problems, thought problems, attention problems and showed more rule-breaking behaviour than typically developing children, whilst the preschool children with MPS-IH only demonstrated significantly more attention and internalising problems. This is interesting given the findings of both Mazefsky et al. (2011), who noted that children with ASD showed a similar pattern of elevated scores on the social, thought and attention syndrome scales of the CBCL, whilst Shapiro et al. (2012) noted a relationship between attention and corpus callosum development in MPS 1H but not in attenuated MPS 1H.

Analyses of the CBCL competence scores showed that school-age children with MPS-IH struggle with the competency areas and skills. This concurs with the findings of Pitt et al. (2009), who suggest that the multiple hospital visits/admissions and limitations set by the residual physical problems due to MPS-IH limit the participation of children with MPS-IH in many everyday activities, a factor not accounted for by the CBCL. The results of the school competence scale are comparable with the known cognitive impairment in children with MPS-IH (Shapiro et al. 2015). With regard to sleep, 57% of parents reported that their children had sleep problems, including bedtime resistance and sleep disordered breathing. The latter is likely to be associated with airway-related problems in MPS-IH (Arn et al. 2015).

The parents of children with MPS-IH did not report experiencing stress levels significantly higher than parents of the normative sample, although 26% scored in the clinical range on the PSI-SF. MPS-IH is diagnosed in the first few months of life but all the children in the current

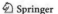

study had already received HCT; it possible that the parents were coping at this stage, or that they had habituated to the stress after having coped with it over a number of years. Alternatively, the parents might find it difficult to admit their stress.

Limitations

The study was limited by the absence of a control group and also because both the SRS and the CBCL measures required using separate forms for younger and older age groups. Although this allows a wider age range to be studied, it necessitated splitting the data, resulting in an overly small sample for the younger group being used in some of the analyses.

Research Implications

The current study adds to the growing body of research indicating that social impairment is more common in developmental genetic disorders. Comparable SRS scores have been observed, for example, in Neurofibromatosis type 1 (NF1) (Garg et al. 2013; Plasschaert et al. 2015) and Turner Syndrome (Lepage et al. 2013). It would be informative to use either of these as a comparison group for the MPS-IH group, as they share the characteristics of physical disability and, in the case of NF1, cognitive impairment. A question for further study is the relationship between social impairment and intellectual disability (Moss and Howlin 2009).

Clinical Implications

Almost a quarter of children with MPS-IH scored in the severe range of the SRS, suggesting clinical-level problems, and fewer than half had scores in the normal range. It is important to recognise this in clinical practice and when planning support for children and families, with timely referrals for ASD assessments. This may bring extra help and resources at school and help to understand hitherto strange or unpredictable behaviours. Similarly, clinicians should be aware that about a third of children with MPS-IH may struggle with social interactions and require help even if they do not reach ASD criteria. The presence of social difficulties should not be overlooked because the children have an MPS-IH diagnosis (diagnostic overshadowing (Dykens 2007)). It is necessary to consider social impairment as children are followed up through childhood and into adolescence, since social demands change with age. Findings from the CBCL suggest that the behaviour of children with MPS-IH can be more difficult to manage and

awareness of this may help parents to understand and accept such behaviours. The presence of specific attentional problems merits further neuropsychological investigation given the potential negative impact on learning. Finally, it is important to investigate the sleep of children with MPS-IH further, as sleep problems appear relatively common in children with MPS-IH. Further research using, for example, actigraphy could differentiate behavioural sleep problems, sleep apnea and airway disease. Additional studies would inform clinical interventions and ensure that sleep problems are not overlooked as merely being typical in childhood.

Synopsis

Children with MPS-IH have problems with social functioning, attention and various competence areas, as rated by their parents.

Contributions of Authors

All authors made substantial contributions to the conception, design and interpretation of the data reported in this chapter. AL was mainly responsible for the acquisition of data, analysis and drafting of the chapter. All authors contributed substantially to the revision of the chapter for intellectual content and all authors provided their final approval of the version to be published.

Dougal Hare acts as guarantor for the chapter, accepts full responsibility for the work and/or the conduct of the study, had access to the data and controlled the decision to publish.

Competing Interests

The authors have no competing interests to declare.

Funding

This review is unfunded as it forms a part of the first author's Clinical Psychology doctorate degree.

Ethical Approval

This study was approved by the North West Greater Manchester Central Research Ethics Committee (15/NW/00/77).

References

Abidin RR (1995) Parenting Stress Index, short form, 3rd edn. Psychological Assessment Resource, Odessa

Achenbach TM, Rescorla LA (2001) Manual for the ASEBA school-age forms & profiles. University of Vermont, Research Center for Children, Youth, & Families, Burlington

Aldenhoven M, Wynn RF, Orchard PJ et al (2015) Long-term outcome of Hurler syndrome patients after hematopoietic cell transplantation: an international multicenter study. Blood 125:2164–2172

Arn P, Bruce IA, Wraith JE, Travers H, Fallet S (2015) Airway-related symptoms and surgeries in patients with Mucopolysaccharidosis I. Ann Otol Rhinol Laryngol 124:198–205

Bax MC, Colville GA (1995) Behaviour in mucopolysaccharide disorders. Arch Dis Child 73:77–81

Bjoraker KJ, Delaney K, Peters C, Krivit W, Shapiro EG (2006) Long-term outcomes of adaptive functions for children with mucopolysaccharidosis I (Hurler syndrome) treated with hematopoietic stem cell transplantation. J Dev Behav Pediatr 27:290–296

Colletti CJ, Wolfe-Christensen C, Carpentier MY et al (2008) The relationship of parental overprotection, perceived vulnerability, and parenting stress to behavioral, emotional, and social adjustment in children with cancer. Pediatr Blood Cancer 51:269–274

Constantino J (2012) The social responsiveness scale, 2nd edn. Western Psychological Services, Los Angeles

Constantino JN, Todd RD (2003) Autistic traits in the general population: a twin study. Arch Gen Psychiatry 60:524–530

Cousino MK, Hazen RA (2013) Parenting stress among caregivers of children with chronic illness: a systematic review. J Pediatr Psychol 38:809–828

D'Aco K, Underhill L, Rangachari L et al (2012) Diagnosis and treatment trends in mucopolysaccharidosis I: findings from the MPS I Registry. Eur J Pediatr 171:911–919

Driscoll KA, Johnson SB, Barker D et al (2010) Risk factors associated with depressive symptoms in caregivers of children with type 1 diabetes or cystic fibrosis. J Pediatr Psychol 35:814–822

Dykens EM (2007) Psychiatric and behavioral disorders in persons with Down syndrome. Ment Retard Dev Disabil Res Rev 13:272–278

Eisengart JB, Rudser KD, Tolar J et al (2013) Enzyme replacement is associated with better cognitive outcomes after transplant in Hurler syndrome. J Pediatr 162:375–380.e1

Garg S, Lehtonen A, Huson SM et al (2013) Autism and other psychiatric comorbidity in neurofibromatosis type 1: evidence from a population-based study. Dev Med Child Neurol 55:139–145

Krivit WJ, Henslee-Downey J, Cowan M et al (1995) Survival in Hurler's disease following bone marrow transplantation in 84 patients. Bone Marrow Transplant 15:S182–S185

Lepage J-F, Dunkin B, Hong DS, Reiss AL (2013) Impact of cognitive profile on social functioning in prepubescent females with Turner syndrome. Child Neuropsychol 19:161–172

Mahon LV, Lomax M, Grant S et al (2014) Assessment of sleep in children with mucopolysaccharidosis type III. PLoS One 9: e84128

Mazefsky CA, Anderson R, Conner CM, Minshew N (2011) Child behavior checklist scores for school-aged children with autism: preliminary evidence of patterns suggesting the need for referral. J Psychopathol Behav Assess 33:31–37

Moore D, Connock MJ, Wraith E, Lavery C (2008) The prevalence of and survival in Mucopolysaccharidosis I: Hurler, Hurler-Scheie and Scheie syndromes in the UK. Orphanet J Rare Dis 3:24

Moss J, Howlin P (2009) Autism spectrum disorders in genetic syndromes: implications for diagnosis, intervention and understanding the wider autism spectrum disorder population. J Intellect Disabil Res 53:852–873

Owens JA, Spirito A, McGuinn M (2000) The Children's Sleep Habits Questionnaire (CSHQ): psychometric properties of a survey instrument for school-aged children. Sleep 23:1043–1051

Pitt C, Lavery C, Wager N (2009) Psychosocial outcomes of bone marrow transplant for individuals affected by Mucopolysaccharidosis I Hurler Disease: patient social competency. Child Care Health Dev 35:271–280

Plasschaert E, Descheemaeker MJ, Van Eylen L, Noens I, Steyaert J, Legius E (2015) Prevalence of autism spectrum disorder symptoms in children with neurofibromatosis type 1. Am J Med Genet B Neuropsychiatr Genet 168B:72–80

Quine L (1991) Sleep problems in children with mental handicap. J Ment Defic Res 35(Pt 4):269–290

Quine L (1992) Severity of sleep problems in children with severe learning difficulties: description and correlates. J Community Appl Soc Psychol 2:247–268

Shapiro E, Evren Guler O, Rudser K, Delaney K, Bjoraker K, Whitley C, Tolar J (2012) An exploratory study of brain function and structure in mucopolysaccharidosis type I: long term observations following hematopoietic cell transplantation (HCT). Mol Genet Metab 107:116–121

Shapiro EG, Nestrasil I, Rudser K et al (2015) Neurocognition across the spectrum of mucopolysaccharidosis type I: age, severity, and treatment. Mol Genet Metab 116:61–68

Wiggs L, Stores G (2001) Behavioural treatment for sleep problems in children with severe intellectual disabilities and daytime challenging behaviour: effect on mothers and fathers. Br J Health Psychol 6:257–269

JIMD Reports
DOI 10.1007/8904_2017_48

Mitochondrial Encephalopathy and Transient 3-Methylglutaconic Aciduria in ECHS1 Deficiency: Long-Term Follow-Up

Irene C. Huffnagel · Egbert J. W. Redeker ·
Liesbeth Reneman · Frédéric M. Vaz ·
Sacha Ferdinandusse · Bwee Tien Poll-The

Received: 07 April 2017 / Revised: 05 July 2017 / Accepted: 07 July 2017 / Published online: 29 July 2017
© Society for the Study of Inborn Errors of Metabolism (SSIEM) 2017

Abstract We report the major diagnostic challenge in a female patient with signs and symptoms suggestive of an early-onset mitochondrial encephalopathy. Motor and cognitive development was severely delayed and brain MRI showed signal abnormalities in the putamen and caudate nuclei. Metabolic abnormalities included 3-methylglutaconic aciduria and elevated lactate levels in plasma and cerebrospinal fluid, but were transient. Whole exome sequencing at the age of 25 years finally revealed compound heterozygous mutations c.[229G>C];[563C>T], p.[Glu77Gln];[Ala188Val] in the *ECHS1* gene. Activity of short-chain enoyl-CoA hydratase, a mitochondrial enzyme encoded by the *ECHS1* gene, was markedly decreased in lymphocytes. Retrospective urine analysis confirms that elevated levels of *S*-(2-carboxypropyl)cysteamine, *S*-(2-carboxypropyl)cysteine, and *N*-acetyl-*S*-(2-carboxypropyl)cysteine can be a diagnostic clue in the disease spectrum of *ECHS1* mutations.

Communicated by: Robin Lachmann, PhD FRCP

I.C. Huffnagel · B.T. Poll-The (✉)
Department of Paediatric Neurology, Emma Children's Hospital, Academic Medical Center, Meibergdreef 9, 1105 AZ Amsterdam, The Netherlands
e-mail: b.t.pollthe@amc.uva.nl

E.J.W. Redeker
Department of Clinical Genetics, Academic Medical Center, Meibergdreef 9, 1105 AZ Amsterdam, The Netherlands

L. Reneman
Department of Radiology, Academic Medical Center, Meibergdreef 9, 1105 AZ Amsterdam, The Netherlands

F.M. Vaz · S. Ferdinandusse
Laboratory Genetic Metabolic Diseases, Academic Medical Center, Meibergdreef 9, 1105 AZ Amsterdam, The Netherlands

Introduction

Short-chain enoyl-CoA hydratase (SCEH, also known as crotonase, EC 4.2.1.17), which is encoded by the *ECHS1* gene (OMIM no. 602292), has a broad substrate specificity and is involved in valine and isoleucine metabolism as well as in mitochondrial β-oxidation of short-chain and medium-chain fatty acids (Wanders et al. 2012). Deficiency of this mitochondrial enzyme has been associated with an encephalopathy similar to Leigh syndrome, in some accompanied by cardiac defects, optic abnormalities, epilepsy, and paroxysmal exercise-induced dystonia. The reported patients show various symptoms and biochemical abnormalities (Peters et al. 2014; Ferdinandusse et al. 2015; Haack et al. 2015; Sakai et al. 2015; Tetreault et al. 2015; Yamada et al. 2015; Ganetzky et al. 2016; Nair et al. 2016; Olgiati et al. 2016; Bedoyan et al. 2017; Al Mutairi et al. 2017; Mahajan et al. 2017).

Here, we report the severe neurological course of a 26-year-old female patient with transient metabolic abnormalities, including 3-methylglutaconic aciduria and elevated lactate levels in plasma and cerebrospinal fluid (CSF). The patient had compound heterozygous mutations, c.[229G>C];[563C>T], p.[Glu77Gln];[Ala188Val] (the latter being novel) in the *ECHS1* gene.

Case Report

The female patient is the first child of non-consanguineous Dutch parents who was born after an uncomplicated pregnancy and delivery with a birth weight of 2.81 kg (10th percentile). The presenting symptom was wandering eye movements at 6 weeks of age with a horizontal nystagmus. Although ophthalmological examination, electroretinography, and visual evoked potentials were normal at first, optical atrophy was noted at the age of 4 years with a visual acuity of 20/100 Snellen equivalent.

Maximum motor development was achieved at 3 months of age with head balance and grasping near objects. Choreoathetosis progressed until the age of 4 but has slowly been ameliorating since. Cognitive development has remained limited to laughing and babbling. To date, at 26 years of age, she shows a spastic tetraparesis and contractures of all major joints with almost no voluntary movements and dystonia during excitement. Visual acuity has diminished to inconsistent light perception. Hearing seems to be intact. Heart ultrasound and an ECG were normal at the age of 20 months. No clinical symptoms and signs of cardiac disease have developed since.

Brain MRI showed mild dilatation of the ventricles with bilateral signal abnormalities on T2-weighted images in the putamen and caudate nuclei at 1 year of age. At the age of 4, atrophy was generalized including basal ganglia and vermis cerebelli superior with signal abnormalities that had progressed to the globi pallidi. No lactate peak was seen on MRS. At 12 years of age atrophy had progressed even further, the corpus callosum was thin, and myelination was delayed (Fig. 1a–i). Repeated EEGs showed no epileptiform activity.

Lactate levels in blood (1.6–4.9 mmol/L; reference range (RR): 0–2.0 mmol/L) were elevated until the age of 7 years, while pyruvate levels were normal. Lactate levels in cerebrospinal fluid (CSF) were also repeatedly elevated (3.2–4.4 mmol/L; RR: 0–2.3 mmol/L) in the first 5 years of life with a marginally elevated pyruvate level (142 μmol/L; RR: 0–130 μmol/L). Analysis of organic acids in urine revealed persistent mild elevations of 3-methylglutaconic acid (22–34 μmol/mmol creatinine; RR: 0–19 μmol/mmol creatinine) until 5 years of age. Levels of 3-methylglutaric acid were slightly increased (7 μmol/mmol creatinine; RR: 0.9–4.5 μmol/mmol creatinine) when the girl was 2 years old and normalized afterwards. Additional organic acid analysis in CSF showed an increase in 3-hydroxyisovaleric acid (15 μmol/L, RR: 1–4 μmol/L) at 2 years of age. This metabolite was also elevated in urine upon leucine-loading (100 mg/kg). Urinary analysis of amino acids was repeatedly normal. Biotinidase activity level in plasma, glutaryl-CoA-dehydrogenase activity in lymphocytes, and 3-methylglutaconyl CoA hydratase activity in fibroblasts were all normal. Holocarboxylase synthetase deficiency was excluded with fibroblast enzyme analysis. A muscle biopsy at 2 years of age revealed no abnormalities in oxidative phosphorylation. Strikingly, even though this patient was severely neurologically affected at 23 years, metabolic profiling, including amino acids, acylcarnitines, and organic acids was normal.

Whole exome sequencing (WES) at 25 years of age revealed compound heterozygous mutations c.[229G>C]; [563C>T], p.[Glu77Gln];[Ala188Val] in the *ECHS1* gene. Mutation analysis by WES confirmed maternal inheritance of c.[229G>C], p.[Glu77Gln] and paternal inheritance of c. [563C>T], p.[Ala188Val]. Activity of SCEH was markedly decreased in lymphocytes (<31 nmol/(min.mg); RR: 101–218 nmol/(min.mg)). Retrospective analysis of metabolites known to be elevated in SCEH deficiency in urine (Peters et al. 2014) showed increased levels of *S*-(2-carboxypropyl)cysteamine, *S*-(2-carboxypropyl)cysteine, and *N*-acetyl-*S*-(2-carboxypropyl)cysteine in our patient (Fig. 1j).

Discussion

The progressive psychomotor retardation, mild 3-methylglutaconic aciduria, and elevated lactate levels in plasma and CSF were highly suggestive for a mitochondrial encephalopathy, which was supported by bilateral signal abnormalities in the basal ganglia on MRI. The increased urinary excretion of 3-methylglutaconic acid was considered an important diagnostic clue, but a muscle biopsy, biotinidase activity level in plasma, glutaryl-CoA-dehydrogenase activity in lymphocytes, and 3-methylglutaconyl CoA hydratase activity in fibroblasts were all normal. In lack of an identified causative disorder, the diagnosis remained unspecified 3-methylglutaconic aciduria for years.

Surprisingly, despite the severe neurological clinical picture, metabolite abnormalities decreased and almost normalized as she got older. Finally, at 25 years of age WES revealed mutations in the *ECHS1* gene, with concomitant decrease in SCEH activity in lymphocytes.

The evolution of the phenotype in this patient highlights the major diagnostic challenge clinicians can face in the diagnosis of the newly recognized disease spectrum of *ECHS1* mutations. The differential diagnosis of mild 3-methylglutaconic aciduria is long and diverse. This transient biochemical abnormality probably was aspecific and due to mitochondrial dysfunction in general (Wortmann et al. 2013). However, in patients with an early-onset severe mitochondrial encephalopathy and absent differentiating biochemical abnormalities, cysteamine/cysteine derivatives should be measured in urine as elevated levels of *S*-(2-carboxypropyl)cysteamine, *S*-(2-carboxypropyl)cysteine, and *N*-acetyl-*S*-(2-carboxypropyl)cysteine can be a diagnostic clue. The urinary levels in our patient were similar to previously reported cases (Peters et al. 2014; Ferdinandusse et al. 2015; Yamada et al. 2015; Olgiati et al. 2016), but not as high as in a severely affected patient that was previously described by Ferdinandusse et al. (2015) (Fig. 1j).

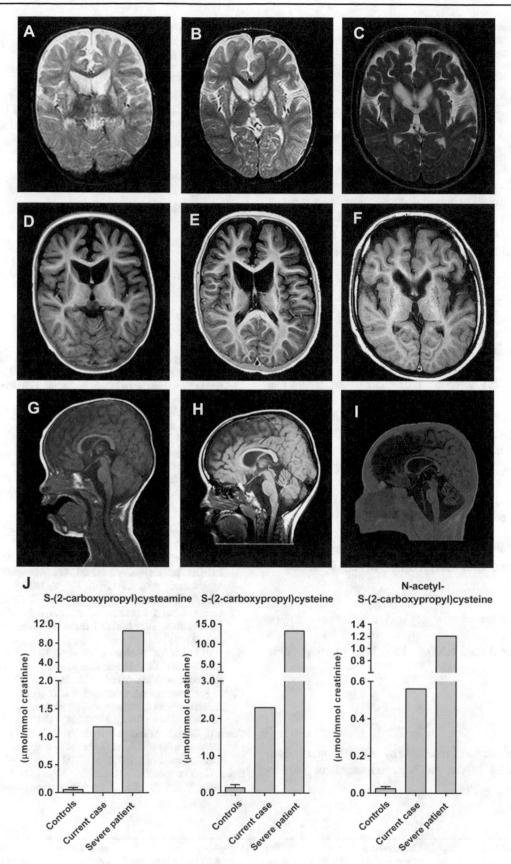

Fig. 1 Brain MRI at age 1, 4, 12 years and metabolite analysis. (**a, d, g**) Brain MRI at age 1 year. (**b, e, h**) Brain MRI at age 4 years. (**c, f, i**) Brain MRI at age 12 years. (**a–c**) Axial T2-weighted images. (**d–f**) Axial T1-weighted images. (**g–i**) Sagittal T1-weighted images.

Acknowledgements We thank Dr. Alberto Burlina (University of Padua, Italy) for providing a urine sample from a previously reported *ECHS1* case for comparison.

Take-Home Message

Elevated levels of *S*-(2-carboxypropyl)cysteamine, *S*-(2-carboxypropyl)cysteine, and *N*-acetyl-*S*-(2-carboxypropyl) cysteine can be a diagnostic clue towards the disease spectrum of *ECHS1* mutations in patients with an early-onset and severe mitochondrial encephalopathy who may survive into adulthood and have transient metabolic abnormalities including 3-methylglutaconic aciduria and elevated lactate levels in plasma and cerebrospinal fluid.

Contributions of Individual Authors

Irene C. Huffnagel: study design, data interpretation, writing manuscript.

Dr. Redeker: analysis and interpretation of genomic array data, critical revision of manuscript for intellectual content.

Dr. Reneman: MRI analysis, critical revision of manuscript for intellectual content.

Dr. Vaz: metabolite analysis, data analysis and interpretation, critical revision of manuscript for intellectual content.

Dr. Ferdinandusse: metabolite analysis, data analysis and interpretation, critical revision of manuscript for intellectual content.

Prof. Dr. Poll-The: study concept, design and supervision, patient care, data interpretation, writing manuscript.

Article Guarantor

Prof Dr. Bwee Tien Poll-The, MD, PhD (corresponding author).

Funding

This research did not receive any specific grant from funding agencies in the public, commercial, or not-for-profit sectors.

Compliance with Ethics Guidelines

Conflict of Interest

Irene C. Huffnagel, Egbert J. W. Redeker, Liesbeth Reneman, Frédéric M. Vaz, Sacha Ferdinandusse, and Bwee Tien Poll-The declare that they have no conflict of interest.

Ethics Approval

Not applicable.

Patient Consent Statement

Informed consent was obtained and available upon request.

References

Al Mutairi F, Shamseldin HE, Alfadhel M, Rodenburg RJ, Alkuraya FS (2017) A lethal neonatal phenotype of mitochondrial short-chain enoyl-CoA hydratase-1 deficiency. Clin Genet 91:629–633

Bedoyan JK, Yang SP, Ferdinandusse S et al (2017) Lethal neonatal case and review of primary short-chain enoyl-CoA hydratase (SCEH) deficiency associated with secondary lymphocyte pyruvate dehydrogenase complex (PDC) deficiency. Mol Genet Metab 120:342–349

Ferdinandusse S, Friederich MW, Burlina A et al (2015) Clinical and biochemical characterization of four patients with mutations in ECHS1. Orphanet J Rare Dis 10:79

Ganetzky RD, Bloom K, Ahrens-Nicklas R et al (2016) ECHS1 deficiency as a cause of severe neonatal lactic acidosis. JIMD Rep 30:33–37

Haack TB, Jackson CB, Murayama K et al (2015) Deficiency of ECHS1 causes mitochondrial encephalopathy with cardiac involvement. Ann Clin Transl Neurol 2:492–509

Mahajan A, Constantinou J, Sidiropoulos C (2017) ECHS1 deficiency-associated paroxysmal exercise-induced dyskinesias: case presentation and initial benefit of intervention. J Neurol 264:185–187

Nair P, Hamzeh AR, Mohamed M, Malik EM, Al-Ali MT, Bastaki F (2016) Novel ECHS1 mutation in an Emirati neonate with severe metabolic acidosis. Metab Brain Dis 31:1189–1192

Olgiati S, Skorvanek M, Quadri M et al (2016) Paroxysmal exercise-induced dystonia within the phenotypic spectrum of ECHS1 deficiency. Mov Disord 31(7):1041–1048

Peters H, Buck N, Wanders R et al (2014) ECHS1 mutations in Leigh disease: a new inborn error of metabolism affecting valine metabolism. Brain 137:2903–2908

Sakai C, Yamaguchi S, Sasaki M, Miyamoto Y, Matsushima Y, Goto Y (2015) ECHS1 mutations cause combined respiratory

---

Fig. 1 (continued) Initial signal abnormalities are limited to the putamen and caudate nuclei, but progress to the globi pallidi. Atrophy is more generalized at follow-up, including involvement of the vermis cerebelli. (**j**) Levels of *S*-(2-carboxypropyl)cysteamine, *S*-(2-carboxypropyl)cysteine, and *N*-acetyl-*S*-(2-carboxypropyl)cysteine in urine measured by tandem mass spectrometry at 23 years of age compared to five healthy controls and one of the severe *ECHS1* cases published by Ferdinandusse et al. (2015)

chain deficiency resulting in Leigh syndrome. Hum Mutat 36:232–239

Tetreault M, Fahiminiya S, Antonicka H et al (2015) Whole-exome sequencing identifies novel ECHS1 mutations in Leigh syndrome. Hum Genet 134:981–991

Wanders RJ, Duran M, Loupatty FJ (2012) Enzymology of the branched-chain amino acid oxidation disorders: the valine pathway. J Inherit Metab Dis 35:5–12

Wortmann SB, Duran M, Anikster Y et al (2013) Inborn errors of metabolism with 3-methylglutaconic aciduria as discriminative feature: proper classification and nomenclature. J Inherit Metab Dis 36:923–928

Yamada K, Aiba K, Kitaura Y et al (2015) Clinical, biochemical and metabolic characterisation of a mild form of human short-chain enoyl-CoA hydratase deficiency: significance of increased N-acetyl-S-(2-carboxypropyl)cysteine excretion. J Med Genet 52:691–698

JIMD Reports
DOI 10.1007/8904_2017_49

RESEARCH REPORT

Glutaric Aciduria Type 3: Three Unrelated Canadian Cases, with Different Routes of Ascertainment

Paula J. Waters · Thomas M. Kitzler ·
Annette Feigenbaum · Michael T. Geraghty ·
Osama Al-Dirbashi · Patrick Bherer ·
Christiane Auray-Blais · Serge Gravel ·
Nathan McIntosh · Komudi Siriwardena ·
Yannis Trakadis · Catherine Brunel-Guitton ·
Walla Al-Hertani

Received: 28 April 2017 / Revised: 23 June 2017 / Accepted: 13 July 2017 / Published online: 02 August 2017
© Society for the Study of Inborn Errors of Metabolism (SSIEM) 2017

Communicated by: Georg Hoffmann

Electronic supplementary material: The online version of this
chapter (doi:10.1007/8904_2017_49) contains supplementary
material, which is available to authorized users.

P.J. Waters (✉) · P. Bherer · C. Auray-Blais · S. Gravel
Division of Medical Genetics, Departments of Pediatrics and Medical
Biology, University of Sherbrooke Hospital Centre (CHUS),
Sherbrooke, QC, Canada
e-mail: Paula.J.Waters@USherbrooke.ca

T.M. Kitzler · Y. Trakadis · W. Al-Hertani
Department of Medical Genetics, McGill University Health Centre
(MUHC), Montreal, QC, Canada

A. Feigenbaum · K. Siriwardena
Division of Clinical and Metabolic Genetics, The Hospital for Sick
Children and University of Toronto, Toronto, ON, Canada

A. Feigenbaum
Division of Genetics, Department of Pediatrics, University of
California, San Diego, CA, USA

M.T. Geraghty · O. Al-Dirbashi · N. McIntosh
Newborn Screening Ontario, Children's Hospital of Eastern Ontario
(CHEO), Ottawa, ON, Canada

O. Al-Dirbashi
College of Medicine and Health Sciences, United Arab Emirates
University, Al Ain, UAE

K. Siriwardena
Department of Medical Genetics, University of Alberta Hospital,
Edmonton, AB, Canada

C. Brunel-Guitton
Division of Medical Genetics, Department of Paediatrics, Sainte-
Justine Hospital and University of Montreal, Montreal, QC, Canada

W. Al-Hertani
Departments of Medical Genetics and Paediatrics, Cumming School
of Medicine, Alberta Children's Hospital and University of Calgary,
Calgary, AB, Canada

Abstract Glutaric aciduria type 3 (GA3) is associated with
decreased conversion of free glutaric acid to glutaryl-coA,
reflecting deficiency of succinate-hydroxymethylglutarate
coA-transferase, caused by variants in the *SUGCT*
(*C7orf10*) gene. GA3 remains less well known, characterised and understood than glutaric aciduria types 1 and 2. It
is generally considered a likely "non-disease," but this is
based on limited supporting information, with only nine
individuals with GA3 described in the literature. Clinicians
encountering a patient with GA3 therefore still face a
dilemma of whether or not this should be dismissed as
irrelevant.

We have identified three unrelated Canadian patients
with GA3. Two came to clinical attention because of
symptoms, while the third was identified by a population
urine-based newborn screening programme and has so far
remained asymptomatic. We describe the clinical histories,
biochemical characterisation and genotypes of these individuals. Examination of allele frequencies underlines the
fact that GA3 is underdiagnosed. While one probable factor
is that some GA3 patients remain asymptomatic, we highlight other plausible reasons whereby this diagnosis might
be overlooked.

Gastrointestinal disturbances were previously reported in
some GA3 patients. In one of our patients, severe episodes
of cyclic vomiting were the major problem. A trial of antibiotic treatment, to minimise bacterial GA production, was
followed by significant clinical improvement.

At present, there is insufficient evidence to define any
specific clinical phenotype as attributable to GA3. However,
we consider that it would be premature to assume that this
condition is completely benign in all individuals at all times.

Introduction

Three distinct types of glutaric aciduria have been described. Glutaric aciduria type 1 (GA1; OMIM 231670; Goodman and Frerman 2001; Boy et al. 2017) is caused by deficiency of glutaryl-CoA dehydrogenase (EC 1.3.8.6), an intramitochondrial flavoprotein required for metabolism of lysine, hydroxylysine and tryptophan. As well as accumulation and increased excretion of glutaric acid (GA), biochemical markers of GA1 include elevations of 3-hydroxyglutaric acid (3HGA), glutaconic acid and glutaryl-carnitine. The natural clinical course of GA1 is characterised by encephalopathic crises, dystonia and dyskinesia, reflecting neuronal degeneration of the striatum.

Glutaric aciduria type 2 (GA2; OMIM 231680; Frerman and Goodman 2001) is caused by decreased activities of multiple acyl-CoA dehydrogenases, reflecting a primary defect in transfer of electrons from these flavoprotein enzymes to the respiratory chain. GA2 is recognised biochemically by characteristic patterns of elevation of several organic acids, acylglycines and acylcarnitines, derived from the various accumulating substrates. Clinical presentations of GA2 reflect, in part, a deficiency of energy generation. However, the pathogenesis of GA2 largely reflects toxicity of accumulated acyl-CoAs and/or of toxic acids derived from alternative metabolism of these acyl-CoAs. The pathogenesis of GA1 likewise reflects toxic consequences of an accumulation of glutaryl-coA and its conversion to toxic acids (Goodman and Frerman 2001). Thus, GA1 and GA2 both represent examples of "CASTOR" (Coenzyme A sequestration, toxicity or redistribution) disorders (Mitchell et al. 2008).

Glutaric aciduria type 3 (GA3, OMIM 231690) is fundamentally distinct from GA1 and GA2, and it is much less well known, characterised and understood than those two conditions. Only nine individuals with GA3 have been described (Bennett et al. 1991; Knerr et al. 2002; Sherman et al. 2008), five asymptomatic, with no single consistent clinical presentation evident in the other four. The observed biochemical phenotype was persistent elevation of GA, notably without elevation of any other markers of GA1 or GA2, and increased GA excretion following lysine loading. The enzyme deficient in GA3 corresponds to an intramitochondrial succinate-hydroxymethylglutarate CoA-transferase (EC 2.8.3.13), encoded by *SUGCT* (originally called *C7orf10*), which converts free GA to glutaryl-CoA (Sherman et al. 2008; Marlaire et al. 2014). While this is probably its main physiological role, several other dicarboxylic acids are good alternative CoA acceptors *in vitro*, glutaryl-CoA and succinyl-CoA are interchangeable CoA donors, and the reaction is easily reversible; together suggesting potential complexity *in vivo* under certain conditions.

GA3 is generally considered a likely "non-disease." However, there is only limited supporting information available. Clinicians encountering a patient diagnosed with GA3 still face the dilemma of whether or not to dismiss this as irrelevant. We therefore describe three unrelated cases, ascertained by different routes, and contribute to the clinical, biochemical and molecular characterisation of this condition.

Patient Descriptions

Patient 1

Patient 1 is an 18-year-old male, born in the province of Ontario, Canada, to non-consanguineous parents of British ancestry. He came to clinical attention at age 22 months with global developmental delay. He had recurrent wheezing episodes in early childhood and admissions for lethargy and unexplained ketonuria/ketoacidosis. There was no history of acute encephalopathy, regression, vomiting episodes or hypoglycemia. MRI at age 2 years showed non-specific periventricular white matter signal change. Growth parameters were unremarkable. He had low-set posteriorly rotated ears, almond shaped eyes, a smallish midfacies with thin upper lip and a sacral dimple.

Qualitative urine organic acid analysis at age 22 months indicated isolated elevation of GA, which was persistent. (Analysis of urine metabolite profiles in recent samples from all patients is described in more detail in the following section, with results in Tables 1 and 2). Results of other metabolic testing, including plasma acylcarnitine and amino acid profiles, were normal. GA1 and GA2 were further excluded by fibroblast studies, respectively by direct enzyme assay and by beta oxidation profiling.

At various times between ages 2 and 7 years, before the diagnosis of GA3 was established and also before the underlying biochemical basis of GA3 was defined, dietary interventions were introduced on an empiric basis, attempting to improve or prevent the recurrent ketotic episodes. A trial of low-fat diet with riboflavin supplementation was changed (following the exclusion of GA2) to a trial of low-protein diet with carnitine supplementation. All such interventions were subsequently discontinued, except carnitine, for which the dose was decreased.

GA3 was diagnosed with the finding of compound heterozygous sequence variants in *SUGCT* (NCBI Reference Sequence NM_001193313.1/NP_001180242.1). The c.1006C>T, p.Arg336Trp variant (previously called c.895C>T, p.Arg299Trp, Sherman et al. 2008) has been reported in other GA3 patients and is deleterious to the protein (Marlaire et al. 2014). The other variant identified

Table 1 Urine organic acids and acylcarnitines

| Patient | Sample | Age | Organic acid profile[a] GC/MS method | | | | | | | Organic acids[a] LC MS/MS | | Acylcarnitines MS/MS | | |
			GA[b]	3HGA[c]	HMG	Ket.	Dic.	Gut	SNS	GA[d]	3HGA[e]	C5DC[f]	C5DC/C5OH[g]	C5DC/C5[h]
1	1-1	16 years	45	5	–	–	–	–	–	65	5.1	0.6	2.1	1.7
2	2-1[i]	4 months	940	7	+	–	–	–	–	NC	NC	NC	2.4	2.5
2	2-2 [i]	6 months	309	0	+	–	–	–	–	NA	NA	NA	NA	NA
2	2-3	9 months	NA	NA	NA	NA	NA	NA	NA	701	4.1	0.4	2.0	1.7
2	2-4	1 year 10 months	153	0	++	–	–	–	–	151	4.7	0.4	2.6	0.2
2	2-5	1 year 10 months	NA	NA	NA	NA	NA	NA	NA	241	5.2	0.5	2.1	0.2
3	3-1[i]	4 weeks	9[j]	0	–	–	–	–	–	NC	NC	NC	1.9	1.8
3	3-2	5 months	91	6	+	–	+	+	+	61	3.0	0.3	3.4	1.8
3	3-3	6 months	48	4	–	–	+	++	+	41	1.2	0.3	3.1	1.2
3	3-4	7 months	144	0	++	++	+	++	+	110	4.3	0.1	2.0	0.9
3	3-5	7 months 3 weeks	166	4	++	++	+	+	+	107	2.1	0.2	4.1	1.7
3	3-6	8 months 2 weeks	393	2	++	+++	+	++	+	NA	NA	NA	NA	NA
3	3-7	1 year 2 months	158	0	–	–	–	–	+	145	4.5	0.7	5.1	1.2
3	3-8	1 year 4 months	38	0	–	–	–	–	–	NA	NA	NA	NA	NA
3	3-9	2 years 9 months	89	0	+	–	–	k	+	111	2.9	0.5	2.6	0.7

GA glutaric acid, *3HGA* 3-hydroxyglutaric acid, *HMG* 3-hydroxy-3-methylglutaric acid, *Ket* ketones, *Dic* dicarboxylic acids, *Gut* acids of probable intestinal origin (including methylmalonic, 3-hydroxypropionic, 4-hydroxyphenyllactic), *SNS* other acids considered secondary or non-specific, *NA* not analysed (specimen not available), *NC* could not be calculated

Concentrations of organic acids other than GA and 3HGA are summarised as follows: – denotes within reference range; + denotes $1\times-3\times$ reference limit; ++ denotes $3\times-10\times$ reference limit; +++ denotes $>10\times$ reference limit

[a] All organic acids are expressed in mmol/mol creatinine. Underlined figures indicate concentrations above reference range

[b] Age-related reference limits for glutaric acid by GC/MS: 12 (age 0–5 months), 22 (5–24 months), 4 (2–12 years), 2 (>12 years)

[c] Age-related reference limits for 3HGA by GC/MS: 10 (0–5 months), 7 (5–24 months), 4 (2–12 years), 5 (>12 years)

[d] Ref. limit: 16

[e] Ref. limit: 7.1

[f] Ref. limit: 5.2 mmol/mol creatinine (Tortorelli et al. 2005; Al-Dirbashi et al. 2011)

[g] Ref. limit (ratio): 10

[h] Ref. limit (ratio): 10

[i] Urine specimen received on filter paper

[j] Retrospective analysis of stored newborn screening filter paper sample

[k] Elevation of lactic acid seen in this specimen only, without elevation of other "gut" markers and without elevation of plasma (L-)lactate, attributed to probable production by gut bacteria

in Patient 1, c.826G>A, p.Val276Ile, is predicted to be deleterious.

Brain MRI, repeated at ages 12 and 16 years, again showed non-specific changes of white matter signal, which were stable from age 12 to age 16. He continues to have attention and impulsivity issues and learning disability, but his cognitive delay is relatively mild and not progressive. He has not had any further ketotic episodes since age 10 years. There are no other clinical concerns.

Patient 2

Patient 2 is a 3-year-old boy, born in the province of Quebec, Canada, to non-consanguineous French-Canadian parents. He came to clinical attention through population urine-based newborn screening. In the Quebec Neonatal Urine Screening Programme (Auray-Blais et al. 2007), an infant's urine sample is collected on filter paper and submitted by parents. Screening is performed on eluted

Table 2 Urine acylglycines

Patient	Sample	Age	Acylglycines[a]			
			Acetylglycine[b]	Propionylglycine[c]	Crotonylglycine[d]	Butyrylglycine[e]
3	3-1[f]	4 weeks	<u>56.51</u>	<u>2.91</u>	<u>11.17</u>	<u>2.74</u>
3	3-2	5 months	<u>50.57</u>	<u>2.27</u>	<u>10.60</u>	<u>3.72</u>
3	3-3	6 months	<u>51.81</u>	<u>3.75</u>	<u>10.39</u>	<u>3.85</u>
3	3-4	7 months	<u>66.83</u>	<u>7.22</u>	<u>18.28</u>	<u>4.90</u>
3	3-5	7 months 3 weeks	<u>71.36</u>	<u>3.56</u>	<u>15.18</u>	<u>3.86</u>
3	3-6	8 months 2 weeks	NA	NA	NA	NA
3	3-7	1 year 2 months	<u>105.95</u>	<u>9.65</u>	<u>2.91</u>	<u>7.22</u>
3	3-8	1 year 4 months	<u>156.45</u>	<u>9.72</u>	<u>2.44</u>	<u>9.49</u>
3	3-9	2 years 9 months	<u>148.00</u>	<u>10.75</u>	<u>6.72</u>	<u>8.27</u>
Ctrl pos ACY1[g]		12 years	<u>81.35</u>	<u>9.66</u>	<u>2.37</u>	<u>3.41</u>

NA not analysed (specimen not available)

Acylglycine profile analysis was performed by an LC-MS/MS method (Bherer et al. 2015) which includes quantitative analysis of 15 acylglycines and semi-quantitative analysis of 6 others. Glutarylglycine analysis is not included in this method

[a] All acylglycines are expressed in mmol/mol creatinine. Underlined figures indicate concentrations above reference range

[b] Age-related reference limits for acetylglycine: 2.55 (age <9 months); 3.13 (age 9 months–8 years)

[c] Age-related reference limits for propionylglycine: 0.15 (age <9 months); 0.15 (age 9 months–8 years)

[d] Age-related reference limits for crotonylglycine: 0.94 (age <9 months); 1.46 (age 9 months–8 years)

[e] Age-related reference limits for butyrylglycine: 0.16 (age <9 months); 0.22 (age 9 months–8 years)

[f] Urine specimen received on filter paper; retrospective analysis of stored newborn screening filter paper sample

[g] "Ctrl pos ACY1" is a positive control urine sample from an individual with aminoacylase 1 deficiency; "Sample 240" provided by the ERNDIM qualitative organic acids (Heidelberg) external quality assurance scheme

samples by thin-layer chromatography, then any samples with apparent substantial elevations of certain organic acids are re-analysed by more quantitative gas chromatography-mass spectrometry (GC-MS) in the biochemical genetics laboratory of CHU Sherbrooke. In two successive screening samples from this infant, GA was elevated, without elevation of markers suggesting GA1 or GA2.

The infant was referred to a metabolic specialist for evaluation. No clinical concerns were identified. Analyses of subsequent urine samples again showed elevation of GA (Table 1). Acylcarnitine profiles were normal in plasma and urine. Analysis of *SUGCT* revealed compound heterozygosity for the known deleterious variant c.1006C>T, p. Arg336Trp, in *trans* with c.625G>A, p.Ala209Thr, which is predicted to be deleterious.

This patient continues to show normal development, without any signs or symptoms of disease, and without any treatment.

Patient 3

Patient 3 is a 4-year-old girl, born in Quebec to French-Canadian parents, who are first cousins. Her urine newborn screening results were negative. She was followed by metabolic specialists because of cyclic vomiting episodes, which began at age 4 months while on breastfeeding, in a

context of gross motor delay, deafness and axial hypotonia. She had a single palmar crease, inverted nipples, frontal bossing, left torticollis and right plagiocephaly. Her head circumference at 6 months had increased to the 90th percentile from the 5th percentile at birth. MRI at age 6 months (Supplementary Fig. 1) showed minimal delayed myelination at the genu of the corpus callosum, and axial CSF space enlargement which raised concern about possible GA1. MR spectroscopy was normal. A repeat MRI at age 1 year was normal.

She continued to have severe episodes with intractable vomiting (10–12 times within a few hours) and dehydration, accompanied by lethargy, metabolic acidosis and ketonuria, with hypoglycemia documented during one episode. These crises occurred at intervals of 2 weeks to 2 months. She was started on L-carnitine (100 mg/kg/day) and riboflavin (100 mg bid).

Plasma acylcarnitine and amino acid profiles were essentially unremarkable. Urine organic acid profiles were somewhat variable; at first they were considered probably non-specific and partly related to gastro-intestinal sources or nutritional status, but GA elevation was noted to be a persistent feature. Profiles were not suggestive of GA1 or GA2. Genetic testing for GA1 (analysis of the *GCDH* gene) was negative. Sequencing of *SUGCT* showed homozygosity for c.1006C>T, p.Arg336Trp, establishing the diagnosis of GA3.

Over time the patient's parents noticed that she had changes in stool quality together with decreased energy and general unwellness in the days immediately prior to each acute episode. This temporal association, recognisable as a recurrent prodrome, prompted clinical suspicion that the episodes could reflect an interplay between the metabolic changes due to GA3 and gut bacterial metabolism. This hypothesis seemed plausible particularly because it is known that free GA can be produced by gut bacteria (Wendel et al. 1995; Kumps et al. 2002). Treatment with the antibiotic metronidazole, to "sterilise" the gut, was therefore introduced on a trial basis (10 mg/kg/day, divided tid, given 10 days per month).

We later noted elevations of several *N*-acetyl-amino acids in urine samples (data not shown). This observation was persistent, being confirmed retrospectively in samples from 5 months of age onwards, and is characteristic of aminoacylase 1 (ACY1) deficiency (Sass et al. 2006; Gerlo et al. 2006). This represented a second unrelated diagnosis for this patient, independent of her diagnosis of GA3. ACY1 deficiency, like GA3, is a condition of uncertain clinical significance; widely considered benign or likely benign, but observed in some patients with non-specific neurological findings (Sass et al. 2007; Tylki-Szymanska et al. 2010). However, it has not been reported in association with episodic metabolic disturbance or cyclic vomiting, therefore did not provide an explanation for this patient's major symptoms.

Other metabolic and genetic testing, for a possible other disorder which could explain the symptoms, especially the cyclic vomiting, has thus far been normal. This has included extensive biochemical workup, mitochondrial DNA sequencing and deletion/duplication testing, molecular analysis for channelopathies and sequencing of the HMG CoA lyase (*HMGCL*) and synthase (*HMGCS2*) genes.

The patient has been doing much better, with only one crisis over the last 18 months, since metronidazole was started. She has sensorineural hearing loss, for which she wears hearing aids. She still has developmental delay, but this is mild and consists of learning difficulties only. There are no other neurological or clinical concerns.

Metabolite Profiles in Urine

Quantitative urine organic acid profiling, by GC-MS following trimethylsilyl derivatisation, was performed at CHUS during clinical investigations of patients 2 and 3. Other investigations for patient 2, at Children's Hospital of Eastern Ontario (CHEO), included analysis of dried urine spots for GA and 3HGA by a liquid chromatography-tandem mass spectrometry (LC-MS/MS) assay (Al-Dirba-shi et al. 2011), with quantification of glutarylcarnitine (C5DC) and associated acylcarnitine ratios by MS/MS (Tortorelli et al. 2005). Patient 3 also had urine acylglycine profiling performed at CHUS by LC-MS/MS (Bherer et al. 2015). Exchanges of available samples later provided results from all methods for all three patients.

Table 1 summarises urine organic acid and acylcarnitine results. Elevation of GA was observed in all urine samples from all patients, except the original newborn screening sample (3-1) from Patient 3. GA values from the GC/MS organic acid profile method and from the dedicated LC-MS/MS method were broadly similar. No sample showed elevation of 3HGA, by either method, nor was 2HGA elevated in any organic acid profile (data not shown). Urine C5DC (expressed relative to creatinine concentration and also as ratios to C5OH and to C5) was consistently normal. These findings were in accord with GA3.

Several samples from Patient 3 showed elevations of organic acids other than GA, including products of gut floral metabolism as well as ketones, dicarboxylic acids and mild elevations of some citric acid cycle metabolites, all supposed secondary to a catabolic state related to vomiting episodes. Her GA levels showed some apparent correlation with variations in her condition, as relatively modest GA elevations were observed at times when the profile was otherwise unremarkable. 3-hydroxy-3-methylglutaric acid (HMG) was elevated in several samples from Patient 3, again tending to correlate with catabolic state. HMG was also somewhat elevated in samples from Patient 2, while his organic acid profiles were otherwise unremarkable.

Acylglycine profiling of urine samples from Patient 3 showed persistent elevations of acetylglycine, propionylglycine, crotonylglycine and butyrylglycine in all specimens, including the original newborn screening filter paper sample (Table 2). Mild elevations of isobutyrylglycine and valerylglycine were also seen in some samples, while all other acylglycines assayed were within reference range (data not shown). No obvious correlations were identified between acylglycine concentrations and concentrations of organic acids in the corresponding samples. Subsequent acylglycine analysis of available specimens from Patients 1 and 2 (samples 1-1, 2-1 and 2-3), by the same method, gave essentially normal results (data not shown). However, analysis of a control sample from an individual with ACY1 deficiency gave a similar profile to those of Patient 3.

Sequence Variants in *SUGCT* (*C7orf10*)

Table 3 summarises the variants identified in our patients, and all previously published variants, with population frequencies from the ExAC database (http://exac.broadinstitute.org).

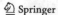

Discussion

We present three cases of GA3; two investigated because of clinical symptoms, the other identified through population screening. There are very few published reports of GA3 patients. Considering observed allele frequencies (Table 3), frequency of GA3 is estimated at ~1/11,000 (European) to ~1/27,000 (Global). This condition is clearly underdiagnosed.

One reason is that some GA3 individuals, perhaps most, remain asymptomatic. GA3 is not detectable by bloodspot acylcarnitine-based newborn screening, as GA3 does not result in accumulation of glutaryl-coA, hence glutarylcarnitine is not elevated. Very few jurisdictions perform urine newborn screening for organic acidemias. In Quebec, only one case of GA3 has been identified by this route in the 16 years (1,161,000 infants screened) since addition of GA1 as a target of the provincial urine screening programme (Auray-Blais et al. 2007); probably because GA was below the detection threshold in most cases.

Some GA3 individuals could have symptoms which are insufficiently specific, severe or persistent to prompt consideration of an inherited disorder. There are other potential reasons why GA3 could be missed, even when "metabolic work-up" is performed. GA excretion levels are variable and often moderate. GA3 is described as presenting with "isolated glutaric aciduria," however this was not always the case with our patients (Table 1); in Patient 3 other acids were often more prominently elevated than GA. Moderate GA elevations are often seen in clinical laboratories; causes or associations (Kumps et al. 2002; Boy et al. 2017) include gut bacterial metabolism and primary or secondary mitochondrial dysfunction. With no known biomarker other than GA, GA3 has been a "diagnosis of exclusion," especially while no genetic or enzymatic test was available. Even with the relevant gene now known, DNA testing is normally only initiated following suspicion based on recognised clinical manifestations or metabolite profiles.

Patient 3 presented with cyclic vomiting. This was true of the first reported GA3 patient (Bennett et al. 1991), while another presented with acute gastroenteritis (Knerr et al. 2002). Both were possibly attributable to, or influenced by, co-existing conditions. A recent abstract (Skaricic et al. 2016) mentions two new patients, one with recurrent vomiting. Intracellular accumulation of free GA, a direct result of GA3, could contribute directly to gastrointestinal disturbances. Our experience with Patient 3 suggests that antibiotic treatment, to minimise bacterial GA production, may be helpful in this context. The significance of interplay between human metabolism and gut microbiome is becoming increasingly recognised, including in patients with inborn errors (Gertsman et al. 2015).

We note that gastrointestinal disturbances are not typical features of either GA1 or GA2, although both conditions are associated with increased GA in body fluids. However, the biochemical basis of GA3 is fundamentally different from that of GA1 or GA2: only in GA3 is the free acid itself a primary substrate of the enzyme, liable to direct accumulation within cells, whereas the elevations of GA observed in blood and urine in GA1 or GA2 arise by a more indirect route via accumulation of glutaryl-coA.

Clinical concerns for Patients 1 and 3 included lethargy, hypotonia and developmental issues. Both had MRI anomalies, albeit minimal and non-specific or transient. Neurological and developmental problems have been described in other GA3 patients (Bennett et al. 1991; Knerr et al. 2002; Skaricic et al. 2016), although some were transient or potentially explicable by other factors.

Patient 3 also has evidence of ACY1 deficiency. We cannot exclude a small possibility that this contributed to her mild developmental delay, but there is no obvious association between ACY1 deficiency and her other symptoms.

There is presently insufficient evidence to define any clinical phenotype as attributable to GA3. However, it would be premature to assume that GA3 is completely benign in all patients at all times. An international collaboration to compile histories of known patients might elucidate common threads, or provide stronger evidence for a lack thereof. Similar considerations apply to ACY1 deficiency.

The biochemical characterisation of GA3 also remains incomplete. For example, elevations of 3-hydroxy-3-methylglutaric acid (HMG) in several samples from two patients (Table 1) were initially discounted as non-specific. HMG is in fact an alternative substrate for C7orf10 *in vitro* (Marlaire et al. 2014), but its *in vivo* significance (if any) in GA3 patients is unknown. Specificity studies with other possible CoA donors and acceptors examined only a few candidate molecules.

The persistently abnormal urine acylglycine profile of Patient 3 was intriguing. There was no obvious link with what is known of the biochemical basis of GA3, and we did not observe similar profiles in our two other GA3 patients. We have, however, seen similar patterns in some other patients in decompensated states, with or without an underlying primary disorder of energy metabolism. It later became apparent that the profile could be attributed in this case to co-existing ACY1 deficiency. N-acetylglycine is a known marker of ACY1 deficiency. It is reasonable to suppose that propionylglycine, crotonylglycine and butyrylglycine (Table 2) are also substrates of ACY1. Broader metabolomic studies on larger groups of GA3 and ACY1-deficient individuals could be worthwhile, particularly in an era where many metabolic enzymes are newly recognised to have additional diverse and significant "moonlighting" roles in other cellular processes (Zschocke 2012; Vilardo and Rossmanith 2015; Boukouris et al. 2016).

Table 3 Sequence variants in *SUGCT* (*C7orf10*) and their frequencies

Variant designations[a]					Allele frequencies[b]	
cDNA	Protein	dbSNP	Identified in this study?	Previously published?	European	Global
c.1006C>T	p.Arg336Trp	rs137852860	Patients 1, 2, 3	Yes[c–e]	0.009295	0.005642
c.826G>A	p.Val276Ile	rs750657344	Patient 1	No	0.00004132	0.00006313
c.625G>A	p.Ala209Thr	rs781200920	Patient 2	No	Not found	0.000008293
c.322C>T	p.Arg108Ter	rs137852862	No	Yes[c]	0.0002758	0.0003234
c.535C>T	p.Arg179Ter	rs137852861	No	Yes[c,e,f]	0.00001498	0.00001656
All five variants (totals of allele frequencies)					0.009627 (1/104)	0.006053 (1/165)

[a] Variant designations (cDNA and protein) used in the present study are based on NCBI Reference Sequence NM_001193313.1/NP_001180242.1
[b] The quoted allele frequencies were obtained from the ExAC (Exome Aggregation Consortium) database (http://exac.broadinstitute.org), which includes 60,706 individuals, of whom approximately half are "European (non-Finnish)"
[c] Sherman et al. (2008)
[d] Variant originally referred to as c.895C>T, p.Arg299Trp
[e] Differences in numbering of some variants, versus the original descriptions by Sherman et al. (2008), are related to the use of a newer reference sequence (also discussed by Marlaire et al. 2014)
[f] Variant originally referred to as c.424C>T, p.Arg142Ter

In summary, we have described three individuals with GA3, two of whom showed clinical symptoms. We propose that this condition may have some clinical significance, if only in a subset of patients or in combination with other factors, and that this possibility warrants investigation.

Acknowledgements We thank the dedicated personnel of the CHUS Biochemical Genetics Laboratory and of the Quebec Provincial Neonatal Urine Screening Programme for logistical, analytical and technical contributions to the laboratory studies.

Synopsis

Glutaric aciduria type 3 may have some clinical significance, if only in a subset of patients or in combination with other factors.

Compliance with Ethics Guidelines

Author Contributions

PJW reviewed and compiled laboratory data and literature, co-ordinated communications with all authors, and wrote much of the manuscript. TMK and WAH initiated a preliminary report of Patients 1 and 3 (poster presentation 204, SSIEM 2014, Kitzler et al., JIMD 37 Suppl. 1:S97), which served as a starting point. TMK, AF, MTG, KS, YT, CBG and WAH (physicians) contributed patient data and clinical descriptions. OAD, PB, CAB and NI (scientists/ analysts) generated and contributed biochemical laboratory results. SG reviewed and discussed molecular genetic data

and population genetic aspects. All authors critically reviewed the first draft and also approved the final manuscript for submission.

Corresponding Author and Guarantor

Paula J. Waters

Conflict of Interest Statements

Paula J. Waters, Thomas M. Kitzler, Annette Feigenbaum, Michael T. Geraghty, Osama Al-Dirbashi, Patrick Bherer, Christiane Auray-Blais, Serge Gravel, Nathan McIntosh, Komudi Siriwardena, Yannis Trakadis, Catherine Brunel-Guitton and Walla Al-Hertani declare that they have no conflict of interest.

Details of Funding

No specific funding was provided for this study.

Ethics Approval

This article does not contain any experimental studies with human or animal subjects performed by any of the authors. Ethics approval was not required for this study.

Patient Consent Statement

Informed consent for publication was obtained from the parents of all patients for whom any identifying information is included in this article.

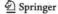

References

Al-Dirbashi OY, Kölker S, Ng D et al (2011) Diagnosis of glutaric aciduria type 1 by measuring 3-hydroxyglutaric acid in dried urine spots by liquid chromatography tandem mass spectrometry. J Inherit Metab Dis 34:173–180

Auray-Blais C, Cyr D, Drouin R (2007) Quebec neonatal mass urinary screening programme: from micromolecules to macromolecules. J Inherit Metab Dis 30:515–521

Bennett MJ, Pollitt RJ, Goodman SI, Hale DE, Vamecq J (1991) Atypical riboflavin-responsive glutaric aciduria, and deficient peroxisomal glutaryl-CoA oxidase activity: a new peroxisomal disorder. J Inherit Metab Dis 14:165–173

Bherer P, Cyr D, Buhas D, Al-Hertani W, Maranda B, Waters PJ (2015) Acylglycine profiling: a new liquid chromatography-tandem mass spectrometry (LC-MS/MS) method, applied to disorders of organic acid, fatty acid and ketone metabolism. J Inherit Metab Dis 38(Suppl 1):S69–S70. Abstract P-028

Boukouris AE, Zervopoulos SD, Michelakis ED (2016) Metabolic enzymes moonlighting in the nucleus: metabolic regulation of gene transcription. Trends Biochem Sci 41:712–730

Boy N, Mülhausen C, Maier EM et al (2017) Proposed recommendations for diagnosing and managing individuals with glutaric aciduria type I: second revision. J Inherit Metab Dis 40:75–101

Frerman FE, Goodman SI (2001) Defects of electron transfer flavoprotein and electron transfer flavoprotein-ubiquinone oxidoreductase: glutaric acidemia type II. In: Scriver CR, Beaudet AL, Sly WS, Valle D (eds) The metabolic and molecular bases of inherited disease, 8th edn. McGraw-Hill, New York, pp 2357–2365

Gerlo E, Van Coster R, Lissens W, Winckelmans G, Meirleir D, Wevers R (2006) Gas chromatographic-mass spectrometric analysis of N-acetylated amino acids: the first case of aminoacylase I deficiency. Anal Chim Acta 571:191–199

Gertsman I, Gangoiti JA, Nyhan WL, Barshop BA (2015) Perturbations of tyrosine metabolism promote the indolepyruvate pathway via tryptophan in host and microbiome. Mol Genet Metab 114:431–437

Goodman SI, Frerman FE (2001) Organic acidemias due to defects in lysine oxidation: 2-ketoadipic acidemia and glutaric acidemia. In: Scriver CR, Beaudet AL, Sly WS, Valle D (eds) The metabolic and molecular bases of inherited disease, 8th edn. McGraw-Hill, New York, pp 2195–2204

Knerr I, Zschocke J, Trautmann U et al (2002) Glutaric aciduria type III: a distinctive non-disease? J Inherit Metab Dis 25:483–490

Kumps A, Duez P, Mardens Y (2002) Metabolic, nutritional, iatrogenic, and artifactual sources of urinary organic acids: a comprehensive table. Clin Chem 48:708–717

Marlaire S, Van Schaftingen E, Veiga-da-Cunha M (2014) C7orf10 encodes succinate-hydroxymethylglutarate CoA-transferase, the enzyme that converts glutarate to glutaryl-CoA. J Inherit Metab Dis 37:13–19

Mitchell GA, Gauthier N, Lesimple A, Wang SP, Mamer O, Qureshi I (2008) Hereditary and acquired diseases of acyl-coenzyme A metabolism. Mol Genet Metab 94:4–15

Sass JO, Mohr V, Olbrich H et al (2006) Mutations in ACY1, the gene encoding aminoacylase 1, cause a novel inborn error of metabolism. Am J Hum Genet 78:401–409

Sass JO, Olbrich H, Mohr V et al (2007) Neurological findings in aminoacylase 1 deficiency. Neurology 68:2151–2153

Sherman EA, Strauss KA, Tortorelli S et al (2008) Genetic mapping of glutaric aciduria, type 3, to chromosome 7 and identification of mutations in C7orf10. Am J Hum Genet 83:604–609

Skaricic A, Zekusic M, Fumic K et al (2016) New symptomatic patients with glutaric aciduria type 3: further evidence of high prevalence of the c.1006C>T (p.Arg336Trp) mutation. J Inherit Metab Dis 39(Suppl 1):S138. Abstract P-275

Tortorelli S, Hahn SH, Cowan TM et al (2005) The urinary excretion of glutarylcarnitine is an informative tool in the biochemical diagnosis of glutaric acidemia type I. Mol Genet Metab 84: 137–143

Tylki-Szymanska A, Gradowska W, Sommer A et al (2010) Aminoacylase 1 deficiency associated with autistic behaviour. J Inherit Metab Dis 33(Suppl 3):S211–S214

Vilardo E, Rossmanith W (2015) Molecular insights into HSD10 disease: impact of SDR5C1 mutations on the human mitochondrial RNase P complex. Nucleic Acids Res 43:5112–5119

Wendel U, Bakkeren J, de Jong J, Bongaerts G (1995) Glutaric aciduria mediated by gut bacteria. J Inherit Metab Dis 18:358–359

Zschocke J (2012) HSD10 disease: clinical consequences of mutations in the HSD17B10 gene. J Inherit Metab Dis 35:81–89

JIMD Reports
DOI 10.1007/8904_2017_51

RESEARCH REPORT

High-Throughput Screen Fails to Identify Compounds That Enhance Residual Enzyme Activity of Mutant N-Acetyl-α-Glucosaminidase in Mucopolysaccharidosis Type IIIB

O. L. M. Meijer · P. van den Biggelaar · R. Ofman · F. A. Wijburg · N. van Vlies

Received: 02 March 2017 / Revised: 19 June 2017 / Accepted: 24 July 2017 / Published online: 24 August 2017
© Society for the Study of Inborn Errors of Metabolism (SSIEM) 2017

Abstract *Background*: In the severe neurodegenerative disorder mucopolysaccharidosis type IIIB (MPSIIIB or Sanfilippo disease type B), deficiency of the lysosomal enzyme N-acetyl-α-glucosaminidase (NAGLU) results in accumulation of heparan sulfate. Patients present with a severe, rapidly progressing phenotype (RP) or a more attenuated, slowly progressing phenotype (SP). In a previous study, residual NAGLU activity in fibroblasts of SP patients could be increased by culturing at 30°C, probably as a result of improved protein folding and lysosomal targeting under these conditions. Chaperones are molecules which influence protein folding and could therefore have therapeutic potential in SP MPSIIIB patients. Here we studied the effects of 1,302 different compounds on residual NAGLU activity in SP MPSIIIB patient fibroblasts including 1,280 approved compounds from the Prestwick Chemical Library.

Methods: Skin fibroblasts of healthy controls, an SP MPSIIIB patient (homozygous for the temperature sensitive mutation p.S612G) and an RP MPSIIIB patient (homozygous for the p.R297* mutation and non-temperature sensitive), were used. A high-throughput assay for measurement of NAGLU activity was developed and validated, after which 1,302 different molecules were tested for their potential to increase NAGLU activity.

Results: None of the compounds tested were able to enhance NAGLU activity.

Conclusions: This high-throughput screen failed to identify compounds that could enhance residual activity of mutant NAGLU in fibroblasts of SP MPSIIIB patients with temperature sensitive mutations. To therapeutically simulate the positive effect of lower temperatures on residual NAGLU activity, first more insight is needed into the mechanisms underlying this temperature dependent increase.

Communicated by: Roberto Giugliani, MD, PhD

Electronic supplementary material: The online version of this chapter (doi:10.1007/8904_2017_51) contains supplementary material, which is available to authorized users.

O.L.M. Meijer · F.A. Wijburg (✉) · N. van Vlies
Department of Pediatric Metabolic Diseases, Emma Children's Hospital and Amsterdam Lysosome Center "Sphinx", Academic Medical Center, Amsterdam, The Netherlands
e-mail: o.l.meijer@amc.uva.nl; f.a.wijburg@amc.uva.nl; naomi.van.vlies@intravacc.nl

O.L.M. Meijer · P. van den Biggelaar · R. Ofman · N. van Vlies
Laboratory of Genetic Metabolic Diseases, Department of Clinical Chemistry, Academic Medical Center, Amsterdam, The Netherlands
e-mail: o.l.meijer@amc.uva.nl; peggyvandenbiggelaar@gmail.com; r.ofman@amc.uva.nl; naomi.van.vlies@intravacc.nl

N. van Vlies
Intravacc, Institute for Translational Vaccinology, Bilthoven, The Netherlands
e-mail: naomi.van.vlies@intravacc.nl

Introduction

In mucopolysaccharidosis type IIIB (MPSIIIB or Sanfilippo disease type B; OMIM#: 252920), deficiency of the lysosomal enzyme N-acetyl-α-glucosaminidase (NAGLU; EC: 3.2.1.50) results in accumulation of the glycosaminoglycan (GAG) heparan sulfate (Muenzer 2011). Patients generally present between the age of 1 and 4 years with a delay in neurocognitive development, predominantly affecting speech and language skills, which is followed by a progressive neurocognitive decline accompanied by behavioral problems (Valstar et al. 2010). There is a wide spectrum of disease severity, ranging from a severe, rapidly progressing phenotype (RP) to a more attenuated, slowly progressing phenotype (SP). Whereas RP patients often die in their late teenage years or early adulthood, patients with an SP phenotype may show a stable developmental impairment for years (Moog et al. 2007; Valstar et al. 2010). No disease modifying treatment is yet available.

Recently, we showed that culturing skin fibroblasts of MPSIIIB patients with an SP phenotype at 30°C significantly increased residual NAGLU activity, probably due to improved protein folding, decreased degradation, and improved targeting to the lysosome (Meijer et al. 2016). Chaperones are molecules that could induce comparable effects and may be considered as potential therapeutic agents for SP MPSIIIB patients. Molecular chaperones, including the heat shock proteins, are endogenous chaperones that play an important role in protein stabilization and are key players in the intracellular protein quality control system (Hartl et al. 2011). Chemical chaperones, on the other hand, are exogenous compounds that stimulate protein folding by nonspecific modes of action (Engin and Hotamisligil 2010; Cortez and Sim 2014), whereas pharmacological chaperones stabilize proteins by more specific binding as they act as ligand to the enzyme or selectively bind a particular native conformation of the protein (Parenti 2009). The use of pharmacological chaperones has been investigated for many diseases affecting protein folding, including LSDs, and several are now in clinical trials (Hollak and Wijburg 2014; Parenti et al. 2015).

Suitable candidates for chaperone therapy in MPSIIIB are 2-acetamido-1,2-dideoxynojirimycin (2AcDNJ) and 6-acetamido-6-deoxycastanospermine, since they were found to be potent inhibitors of purified human NAGLU and its bacterial homolog (Zhao and Neufeld 2000; Ficko-Blean et al. 2008). Another compound of interest is glucosamine. Treatment of cultured fibroblasts from MPS IIIC patients (OMIM#: 252930) with glucosamine partially restored the activity of the deficient enzyme heparan acetyl-CoA:alpha-glucosaminide *N*-acetyltransferase (HGSNAT; EC:2.3.1.78). This could also be the case for MPSIIIB, as NAGLU binds glucosamine residues at the non-reducing end of the GAG chain (Feldhammer et al. 2009; Matos et al. 2014).

Here we aimed to investigate the effects of known chemical and pharmacological chaperones on residual enzyme activity in a MPSIIIB fibroblast cell line in which residual enzyme activity can be increased by culturing at low temperature. Also, we investigated the effect of the 1,280 approved compounds from the Prestwick Chemical Library, which have all proven their safety in humans.

Material and Methods

Cell Culture

Cultured skin fibroblasts of healthy controls, a MPSIIIB patient with an SP phenotype, homozygous for the temperature sensitive missense mutation p.S612G, and of a MPSIIIB patient homozygous for the p.R297* mutation conveying an RP phenotype and previously demonstrated not to be temperature sensitive, were selected for validation of the assay and subsequent compound screen (Meijer et al. 2016). Fibroblasts were cultured in Dulbecco's Modified Eagle's Medium (DMEM) supplemented with 10% Fetal Bovine Serum (FBS) and 100 U/mL penicillin, 100 µg/mL streptomycin, and 250 µg/mL amphotericin at 37°C (unless otherwise stated) in a humidified atmosphere containing 5% CO_2. Before adding FBS to the medium, bovine NAGLU was inactivated by incubation of FBS at 65°C for 35 min. All cell lines were found negative for mycoplasma contamination.

NAGLU Activity Assay

NAGLU activity in protein homogenates of skin fibroblasts was measured according to our previously described method (Meijer et al. 2016). Since this method is unsuitable for screening of a large number of compounds, an assay suitable for high-throughput screening was designed, based on the method described by Mauri et al. (2013). Fluorogenic 4-methylumbelliferyl-2-acetamido-2-deoxy-α-D-glucopyranoside (4MU-α-GlcNAc) (Moscerdam, Oegstgeest, The Netherlands) was used as substrate and dissolved to the required concentration in a 0.1 M citrate 0.2 M phosphate buffer pH 4.3. The assay was started by adding 50 µL reaction mixture (12.5 µL 4MU-α-GlcNAc, 37 µL 0.1 M citrate 0.2 M phosphate buffer pH 3.85 and 0.5 µL 10% Triton-X100) to each well which was incubated at 37°C for different time periods. The reaction was stopped by adding 150 µL 0.2 M sodium carbonate buffer pH 10.5. Fluorescence of released 4-methylumbelliferone was measured with a Fluostar Optima Microplate Reader (BMG Labtech, Ortenberg, Germany), using an excitation and emission wavelength of 360 nm and 450 nm, respectively. NAGLU activity was calculated using a calibration curve of 4-methylumbelliferone (Glycosynth Ltd., Warrington, Cheshire, UK).

Compound Screen

Cells were harvested by trypsinization, counted using a Z™ series Coulter Counter (Beckman Coulter Inc., Brea,

California, United States) and diluted in culture medium to the required concentrations. For each cell line, 100 μL cell suspension per well was plated in black, clear bottom 96-well plates (Greiner Bio-One, Kremsmünster, Austria). Next day, culture medium was replaced with 200 μL culture medium containing one of the small compounds described below and incubated for 5 days following our standard protocol. After 5 days incubation, plates were washed three times with phosphate buffered saline (PBS) and NAGLU activity was measured as described above.

Chemicals

Taurine, D-arginine, L-homoarginine hydrochloride, saccharose, trimethylamine *N*-oxide (TMAO), dimethyl sulfoxide (DMSO $\geq$99.9%), ambroxol, D-glucosamine hydrochloride, *N*-acetylglucosamine, trichostatin A (TSA), bortezomib, and ursodeoxycholic acid (UDCA) were all purchased from Sigma-Aldrich (St. Louis, MO, USA). L-arginine monohydrochloride, trehalose and 4-phenylbutyrate (4-PBA) were from Merck (Darmstadt, Germany), β-alanine from BDH (Analytical Chemicals, VWR International, Radnor, PA, USA), glycerol and betaine were from Arcos Organics (Geel, Belgium), and glycine from Serva Electrophoresis GmbH (Heidelberg, Germany). Tauroursodeoxycholic acid (TUDCA) was from Calbiochem (Merck Millipore, Billerica, MA, USA), 2-acetamido-1,2-dideoxynojirimycin (2AcDNJ) from Bio-connect (Life Sciences, Huissen, The Netherlands), and suberanilohydroxamic acid (SAHA or Vorinostat) from Cayman Chemical Company (Ann Arbor, MI, USA).

The compounds used in our screen were first dissolved in milliQ (Synergy Water Purification System, Merck Millipore, Billerica, MA, USA), sterilized using a 0.45 μm syringe filter (Merck Millipore, Billerica, MA, USA) and diluted in culture medium to the required concentration. Except for UDCA, ambroxol, bortezomib, TSA, and SAHA, for which stock solutions were prepared in DMSO and subsequently diluted in culture medium (final DMSO concentration 1.0%).

The Prestwick Chemical Library (Prestwick Chemical, Illkirch, France) consisted of 1,280 compounds (2 mM stock solutions in DMSO), which were diluted in culture medium to a final concentration of 10 μM (final DMSO concentration 0.5%).

Western Blot Analysis

Cell pellets were dissolved in milliQ supplemented with cOmplete™ protease inhibitor cocktail (Roche, Mannheim, Germany) and disrupted by sonification using a Vibra Cell sonicator (Sonics & Materials Inc., Newtown, CT, USA). Protein concentration was measured in whole cell lysates as

described by Lowry et al. (1951). For Western blot analysis of NAGLU, 50 μg of protein was loaded onto a NuPAGE Novex 4–12% Bis-Tris pre-cast polyacrylamide gel (Invitrogen, Carlsbad, CA, USA) that after electrophoresis was transferred onto an Amersham Protran Nitrocellulose Blotting Membrane by semidry blotting (GE Healthcare Life Sciences, Little Chalfont, UK). Membranes were blocked in 30 g/L bovine serum albumin (Sigma-Aldrich, St. Louis, MO, USA) in 0.1% Tween-20 in PBS (TPBS). Antibodies used were: rabbit anti-NAGLU antibody 1:800 (ab169874; Abcam, Cambridge, UK), mouse anti-β-actin antibody 1:10,000 (Sigma-Aldrich, St. Louis, MO, USA), goat anti-rabbit and donkey anti-mouse antibody 1:10,000 (IRDye 800CW and IRDye 680RD, respectively; LI-COR Biosciences, Lincoln, NE, USA). Primary antibodies were dissolved in TPBS and secondary antibodies in TPBS with Odyssey® blocking buffer and SDS 0.01%. Between antibody incubations membranes were washed five times with TPBS. Blots were analyzed using the Odyssey® CLx Infrared Imaging System (LI-COR Biosciences, NE, USA).

Statistical Analysis

Data analyses were performed using SPSS software for Windows (version 23.0, SPSS Inc., Chicago, IL, USA). A *p*-value of <0.05 was considered statistically significant.

Results

Effects of Culturing at 30°C on Mutant NAGLU

Previously it has been shown that residual activity of NAGLU in fibroblasts of MPSIIIB patients with an SP phenotype can be increased by culturing at 30°C (Meijer et al. 2016). To further investigate the increase in activity of mutant NAGLU at low culture temperature, NAGLU protein and activity levels were determined in control and MPSIIIB fibroblast cell lines after culturing at 37 and 30°C (Fig. 1a). Western blot analysis of fibroblasts from a healthy control cultured at 37°C showed that NAGLU consists of two forms: a precursor form with an apparent molecular weight of 85 kD and a mature form with an apparent molecular weight of 82 kD. In the SP p.S612G MPSIIIB cell line, only the precursor form was detected after culturing at 37°C, whereas after culturing at 30°C both NAGLU forms could be observed. This corresponded with an increase in NAGLU activity from 0.41 nmol mg^{-1} h^{-1} after culturing at 37°C up to 4.06 nmol mg^{-1} h^{-1} after culturing at 30°C (Fig. 1b; NAGLU activity in control fibroblasts cultured at 37°C: 19.71 nmol mg^{-1} h^{-1}). In fibroblasts of the RP p.R297* MPSIIIB patient, no NAGLU

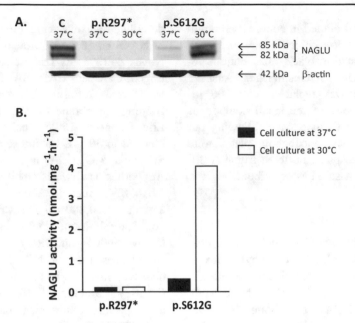

Fig. 1 (**a**) Western blot analysis of NAGLU protein levels and (**b**) corresponding activity levels (nmol mg^{-1} h^{-1}) after culturing MPSIIIB patient and control fibroblasts at 37 and 30°C for 1 week. NAGLU activity was measured as was described previously (Meijer et al. 2016). NAGLU activity in control fibroblasts cultured at 37°C was 19.71 nmol mg^{-1} h^{-1}

protein was present under either of these conditions (measured NAGLU activities: 0.14 and 0.15 nmol mg^{-1} h^{-1} after culturing at 37°C and 30°C, respectively).

Optimization and Validation of the 96-Well NAGLU Assay

Prior to the compound screen, a method suitable for high-throughput applications was developed based on the method described by Mauri et al. (2013) and optimized for incubation time, 4MU-α-GlcNAc substrate concentration and cell density (Supplementary figure 1). Based on these results we decided to use 10,000 cells/well and to measure NAGLU activity after 5 days of culturing using 1 mg/mL 4MU-α-GlcNAc substrate incubated at 37°C for 24 h. Since at present no compound is known that can enhance residual NAGLU activity in MPSIIIB fibroblasts, fibroblasts of a healthy subject were used as a positive control and plated at a density of 2,500 cells/well in each plate. As chaperones only act on missense variants, p. R297* MPS IIIB fibroblasts plated at a density of 10,000 cells/well were included as a negative control. Since this cell line contains a mutation resulting in a premature stop, no protein will be synthesized and no activity was expected to be measured.

Using these conditions, the Z-factor of the assay was determined, which is considered a reliable measure for evaluation and validation of high-throughput screens (Zhang et al. 1999). A calculated Z-factor of 0.69 classified this assay as "excellent."

Effect of Chemical Chaperones

Chemical chaperones are generally divided into two subgroups: the osmolytes and hydrophobic compounds (Cortez and Sim 2014). Several classes of osmolytes were studied: free amino acids and amino acid derivatives (β-alanine, glycine, taurine, D-arginine, L-homoarginine hydrochloride, L-arginine monohydrochloride), carbohydrates (trehalose and saccharose), polyols (glycerol), methyl-amines (betaine and TMAO), and organosulfur compounds (DMSO). In addition the effect of the hydrophobic chaperones 4-PBA and the bile acids UDCA and TUDCA was assessed.

None of the 15 chemical chaperones tested, enhanced NAGLU activity in MPSIIIB fibroblasts after 5 days incubation at different concentrations (Fig. 2a).

Effect of Pharmacological Chaperones, Previously Investigated in LSDs

Pharmacological chaperones previously studied for potential effects in LDSs were assessed and included ambroxol (Maegawa et al. 2009), the proteasome inhibitor bortezomib (Shimada et al. 2011; Macías-Vidal et al. 2014) and the HDAC inhibitors TSA and SAHA (Pipalia et al. 2011). None of these compounds enhanced residual NAGLU activity in p.S612G MPSIIIB fibroblasts (Fig. 2b).

The (N-acetyl)glucosamine inhibitors D-glucosamine, N-acetylglucosamine, and 2AcDNJ, which were previously

A.

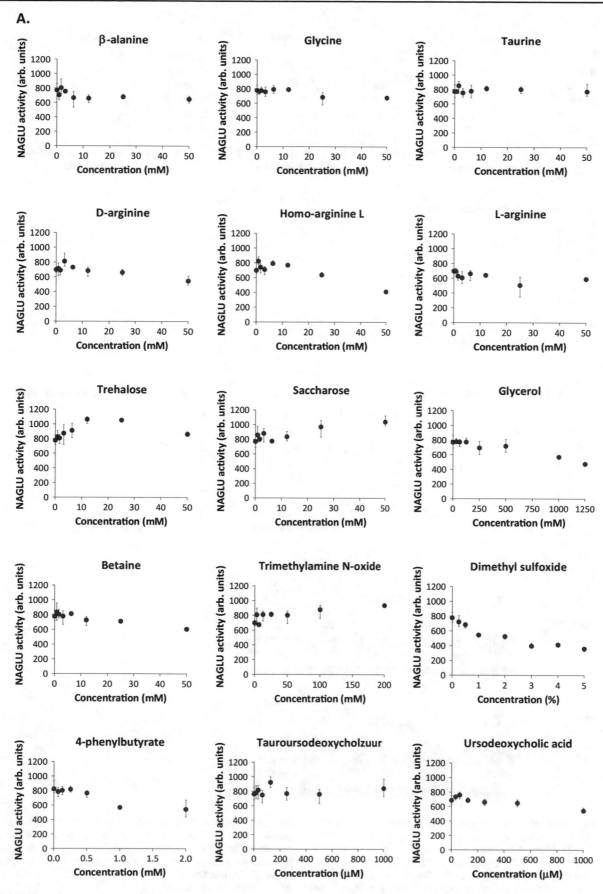

Fig. 2 (continued)

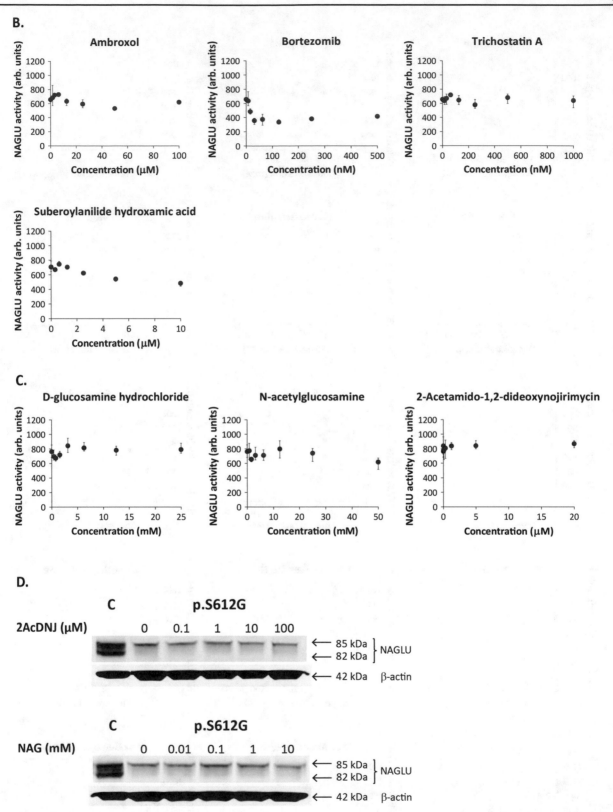

Fig. 2 (**a**) Effect of treatment with different classes of chemical chaperones on residual NAGLU activity in p.S612G MPSIIIB fibroblasts. (**b**) Effect of treatment with pharmacological chaperones used in other protein folding diseases including LDSs, on residual NAGLU activity in p.S612G MPSIIIB fibroblasts. (**c**) Effect of treatment with pharmacological chaperones used in MPS III on residual NAGLU activity in p.S612G MPSIIIB fibroblasts. NAGLU activity levels are shown in fluorescence (arb. units). All compound concentrations were tested in triplicate. Mean ± SD is given. (**d**) Western blot analysis of the effect of treatment with *N*-acetylglucosamine (NAG) and 2AcDNJ for 5 days on NAGLU protein levels in p. S612G MPSIIIB fibroblasts

shown to affect NAGLU and HGSNAT in MPSIIIB and MPS IIIC respectively, were also investigated (Zhao and Neufeld 2000; Ficko-Blean et al. 2008; Feldhammer et al. 2009; Matos et al. 2014). As is shown in Fig. 2c, treatment with these compounds did not lead to significant enhancement of NAGLU activity levels.

To investigate whether any of these compounds did have an effect on protein levels, which, due to a too strong inhibitory effect, may not have resulted in detectable changes in enzyme activity, the effect of N-acetylglucosamine and 2AcDNJ on NAGLU protein was assessed on Western blot (Fig. 2d). Treatment with neither of these compounds led to higher expression of the precursor of NAGLU or the formation of the mature form of the enzyme.

Prestwick Chemical Library

So far none of the compounds tested showed any effect on residual activity of mutant NAGLU. Therefore the Prestwick Chemical Library was tested consisting of 1,280 approved drugs (Fig. 3a). All compounds with a fluorescent signal of 500 arb. units or above the mean background were selected for further analyses. These included the antihypertensive drugs benzamil hydrochloride (PCL-657) and doxazosin mesylate (PCL-858), the anti-osteoporetic drug ibandronate sodium (PCL-1285), the xanthine oxidase inhibitor used for the treatment of gout, allopurinol (PCL-1213), and the antiseptic drug aminacrine (PCL-1717). To validate the results of the screen, MPSIIIB p.S612G fibroblasts were incubated for 5 days with the selected compounds at increasing concentrations. Both ibandronate sodium and allopurinol did not show any significant effect on NAGLU activity (Fig. 3b). For aminacrine, benzamil hydrochloride, and doxasozin mesylate a dose dependent increase in fluorescent signal was observed. However, the same increase in fluorescence was obtained when the assay was repeated in the absence of the 4MU-α-GlcNAc substrate, indicating that there is no actual increase in residual NAGLU activity upon treatment with these compounds.

Discussion

We assessed the effect of 1,302 different molecules on residual enzyme activity in a MPSIIIB patient fibroblast cell line which responded with a significant increase in NAGLU activity when cultured at 30°C instead of 37°C (Meijer et al. 2016). As enzyme activity is related to the efficiency of protein folding, culturing at 30°C may improve folding of the mutant NAGLU enzyme (Fan 2003; Gootjes et al. 2004). Unfortunately, none of the molecules tested in our assay,

including the 1,280 compounds from the Prestwick Chemical Library, were effective.

The observed lack of effect may well be understood if protein misfolding is not, or only to a limited extend, involved in the SP MPSIIIB phenotype and if the observed increase in enzyme activity in fibroblasts cultured at 30°C is due to other mechanisms. Indeed, our observation on Western blot that at 37°C culture conditions only the 85 kDa precursor form of NAGLU is detected while at 30°C also the mature 82 kDa NAGLU protein is observed rather suggests differences in protein synthesis and processing.

The majority of chemical chaperones studied here have remarkable general mechanisms of action and were shown to influence enzymatic activity in other protein folding diseases including LSDs (Maegawa et al. 2009; Pipalia et al. 2011; Shimada et al. 2011; Cortez and Sim 2014; Macías-Vidal et al. 2014). We consider that, if protein misfolding is indeed involved in the MPSIIIB SP phenotype, some effect of these compounds would have been observed. Our observation that more NAGLU specific compounds such as the N-acetylglucosaminidase inhibitors N-acetylglucosamine and 2AcDNJ also lacked effect on NAGLU protein and activity levels further supports the hypothesis that protein misfolding does not play a major role in MPSIIIB. In previous studies the binding capacity of 2AcDNJ has always been assessed using purified NAGLU (Zhao and Neufeld 2000; Ficko-Blean et al. 2008). As NAGLU is synthesized in the rough endoplasmic reticulum (ER), it is possible that these compounds do have the capacity to bind and stabilize mutant NAGLU, but cannot enter the ER in a cell culture model as used here. This may also have blocked potential effects of other compounds tested in this study, although it is unlikely that compounds which do not reach the target protein in vitro would have therapeutic properties in vivo. Thus, despite the promising effects of chaperones in other LSDs such as Fabry disease, this approach may not serve all LSDs as was shown here for MPS IIIB (Hollak and Wijburg 2014; Germain et al. 2016; Hughes et al. 2017).

A limitation of this study is that compounds were tested in one MPSIIIB cell line. Although this cell line was selected because its mutation conveys an SP phenotype and enzyme activity responded favorably to culturing at 30°C, we cannot exclude that this mutation is insensitive to the here tested compounds and that they might have had a positive effect on other mutations. However, allelic heterogeneity in MPSIIIB is large, and it would not be feasible to test all reported mutations (Valstar et al. 2010). A drawback of high-throughput screens in general is that compound libraries are often tested in a limited number of concentrations, so that an effect of any of the compounds at a different concentration cannot be ruled out.

Thus, despite a reliable and robust assay, this high-throughput screen failed to identify compounds that could

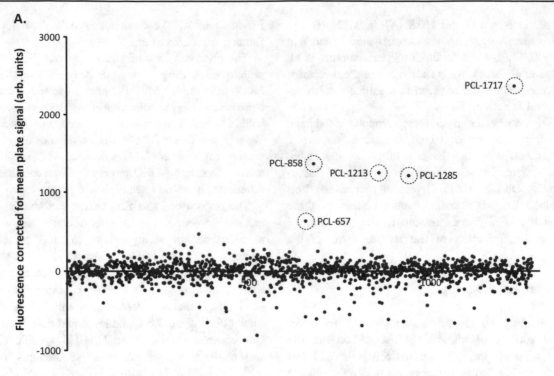

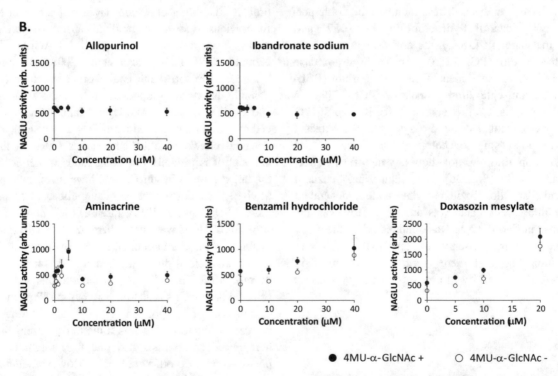

Fig. 3 (**a**) Effect of treatment with compounds from the Prestwick Chemical Library (10 μM) on NAGLU activity in p.S612G MPSIIIB fibroblasts. NAGLU activity levels are shown in fluorescence (arb. units) and were corrected for the mean plate signal. (**b**) Validation of the compounds identified in the high-throughput screen of the

Prestwick Chemical Library in p.S612G MPSIIIB fibroblasts. NAGLU activity levels are shown in fluorescence (arb. units) after incubation with or without 4MU-α-GlcNAc substrate. All compound concentrations were tested in triplicate. Mean ± SD is given

enhance residual activity of mutant NAGLU in fibroblasts of an SP MPSIIIB patient homozygous for a temperature

sensitive mutation. We conclude that to therapeutically simulate the positive effect of lower temperatures on residual NAGLU activity, first more insight is needed into the mechanisms underlying this temperature dependent increase in enzyme activity.

Acknowledgements The authors would like to thank Dr. S. F. van de Graaf of the Tytgat Institute for Liver and Intestinal Research/ Department of Gastroenterology & Hepatology at the Academic Medical Center in Amsterdam, for being so kind to provide the Prestwick Chemical Library to us. This study was funded by grants from the private foundations "Stichting Stofwisselkracht," "Zabawas," "Zeldzame Ziekten Fonds," and "Kinderen en Kansen," the Netherlands.

Take Home Message

High-throughput screen fails to identify compounds that enhance residual enzyme activity of mutant *N*-acetyl-α-glucosaminidase in mucopolysaccharidosis type IIIB.

Author Contributions

O. L. M. Meijer:	Designed and conducted the study, was responsible for data analysis and interpretation and for writing of the article
P. van den Biggelaar:	Assisted in the conduction of the study
R. Ofman:	Assisted in the design and conduction of the study
F. A. Wijburg:	Designed and supervised the study, revised the manuscript
N. van Vlies:	Designed and supervised the study, revised the manuscript

Guarantor for the Article

F. A. Wijburg, MD PhD, Department of Pediatric Metabolic Diseases, Emma Children's Hospital and Amsterdam Lysosome Center "Sphinx," Academic Medical Center, Meibergdreef 9, 1105 AZ Amsterdam, The Netherlands, f.a.wijburg@amc.uva.nl.

Authors Conflict of Interest

O. L. M. Meijer, P. van den Biggelaar, R. Ofman, F. A. Wijburg, and N. van Vlies declare that they have no conflict of interest.

Details of Funding

This study was funded by grants from the private foundations "Stichting Stofwisselkracht," "Zabawas," "Zeldzame Ziekten Fonds," and "Kinderen en Kansen," the Netherlands.

Details of Ethics Approval

No ethics approval was required for this study. This article does not contain any studies with human or animal subjects performed by any of the authors.

Informed Consent

Informed consent for the use of patient fibroblasts was obtained from parents or legal representatives for all patients.

Animal Rights

This article does not contain any studies with animal subjects performed by any of the authors.

References

Cortez L, Sim V (2014) The therapeutic potential of chemical chaperones in protein folding diseases. Prion 8:197–202

Engin F, Hotamisligil GS (2010) Restoring endoplasmic reticulum function by chemical chaperones: an emerging therapeutic approach for metabolic diseases. Diabetes Obes Metab 12:108–115

Fan JQ (2003) A contradictory treatment for lysosomal storage disorders: inhibitors enhance mutant enzyme activity. Trends Pharmacol Sci 24:355–360

Feldhammer M, Durand S, Pshezhetsky AV (2009) Protein misfolding as an underlying molecular defect in mucopolysaccharidosis III type C. PLoS One 4:e7434

Ficko-Blean E, Stubbs KA, Nemirovsky O et al (2008) Structural and mechanistic insight into the basis of mucopolysaccharidosis IIIB. Proc Natl Acad Sci U S A 105:6560–6565

Germain DP, Hughes DA, Nicholls K et al (2016) Treatment of Fabry's disease with the pharmacologic chaperone migalastat. N Engl J Med 375:545–555

Gootjes J, Schmohl F, Mooijer PA et al (2004) Identification of the molecular defect in patients with peroxisomal mosaicism using a novel method involving culturing of cells at 40°C: implications for other inborn errors of metabolism. Hum Mutat 24:130–139

Hartl FU, Bracher A, Hayer-Hartl M (2011) Molecular chaperones in protein folding and proteostasis. Nature 475:324–332

Hollak CE, Wijburg FA (2014) Treatment of lysosomal storage disorders: successes and challenges. J Inherit Metab Dis 37:587–598

Hughes DA, Nicholls K, Shankar SP et al (2017) Oral pharmacological chaperone migalastat compared with enzyme replacement therapy in Fabry disease: 18-month results from the randomised phase III ATTRACT study. J Med Genet 54:288–296

Lowry OH, Rosebrough NJ, Farr AL, Randall RJ (1951) Protein measurement with the Folin phenol reagent. J Biol Chem 193:265–275

Macías-Vidal J, Girós M, Guerrero M et al (2014) The proteasome inhibitor bortezomib reduced cholesterol accumulation in fibroblasts from Niemann-Pick type C patients carrying missense mutations. FEBS J 281:4450–4466

Maegawa GH, Tropak MB, Buttner JD et al (2009) Identification and characterization of ambroxol as an enzyme enhancement agent for Gaucher disease. J Biol Chem 284:23502–23516

Matos L, Canals I, Dridi L et al (2014) Therapeutic strategies based on modified U1 snRNAs and chaperones for Sanfilippo C splicing mutations. Orphanet J Rare Dis 9:180

Mauri V, Lotfi P, Segatori L, Sardiello M (2013) A rapid and sensitive method for measuring N-acetylglucosaminidase activity in cultured cells. PLoS One 8:1–9

Meijer OL, Welling L, Valstar MJ et al (2016) Residual N-acetyl-α-glucosaminidase activity in fibroblasts correlates with disease severity in patients with mucopolysaccharidosis type IIIB. J Inherit Metab Dis 39:437–445

Moog U, van Mierlo I, van Schrojenstein Lantman-de Valk HM et al (2007) Is Sanfilippo type B in your mind when you see adults with mental retardation and behavioral problems? Am J Med Genet C Semin Med Genet 145C:293–301

Muenzer J (2011) Overview of the mucopolysaccharidoses. Rheumatology 50(suppl 5):v4–v12

Parenti G (2009) Treating lysosomal storage diseases with pharmacological chaperones: from concept to clinics. EMBO Mol Med 1:268–279

Parenti G, Andria G, Valenzano KJ (2015) Pharmacological chaperone therapy: preclinical development, clinical translation, and prospects for the treatment of lysosomal storage disorders. Mol Ther 23:1138–1148

Pipalia NH, Cosner CC, Huang A et al (2011) Histone deacetylase inhibitor treatment dramatically reduces cholesterol accumulation in Niemann-Pick type C1 mutant human fibroblasts. Proc Natl Acad Sci U S A 108:5620–5625

Shimada Y, Nishida H, Nishiyama Y et al (2011) Proteasome inhibitors improve the function of mutant lysosomal α-glucosidase in fibroblasts from Pompe disease patient carrying c.546G>T mutation. Biochem Biophys Res Commun 415:274–278

Valstar MJ, Bruggenwirth HT, Olmer R et al (2010) Mucopolysaccharidosis type IIIB may predominantly present with an attenuated clinical phenotype. J Inherit Metab Dis 33:759–767

Zhang JH, Chung TD, Oldenburg KR (1999) A simple statistical parameter for use in evaluation and validation of high throughput screening assays. J Biomol Screen 4:67–73

Zhao KW, Neufeld EF (2000) Purification and characterization of recombinant human α-N-acetylglucosaminidase secreted by Chinese hamster ovary cells. Protein Expr Purif 19:202–211

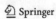

JIMD Reports
DOI 10.1007/8904_2017_52

RESEARCH REPORT

Demographic and Psychosocial Influences on Treatment Adherence for Children and Adolescents with PKU: A Systematic Review

**Emma Medford · Dougal Julian Hare ·
Anja Wittkowski**

Received: 30 August 2016 / Revised: 20 July 2017 / Accepted: 24 July 2017 / Published online: 25 August 2017
© Society for the Study of Inborn Errors of Metabolism (SSIEM) 2017

Abstract Phenylketonuria (PKU) is a rare genetic disorder in which the amino acid phenylalanine cannot be sufficiently metabolised. Although a build-up of phenylalanine causes irreversible cognitive impairment, this can be prevented through a strict, lifelong diet restricted in natural protein. Despite the severe consequences of poor metabolic control, many children and adolescents have phenylalanine levels above their recommended limits. This systematic review was the first to examine studies reporting demographic and/or psychosocial influences on blood phenylalanine levels, with the aim to identify factors that were robustly linked with metabolic control. Four electronic databases were searched, yielding 1,808 articles. Articles were included if they reported a statistical examination of the association between one or more demographic or psychosocial factor(s) and metabolic control (as measured by blood phenylalanine concentration) for children and adolescents with PKU. Twenty-nine studies were selected for inclusion, which examined a range of child, parent and family factors related to blood phenylalanine levels. The most reproducible association was with child age, with metabolic control worsening with increasing age. This suggests that interventions promoting treatment adherence would be particularly beneficial for adolescents. There was a paucity of studies in some areas, and the quality of included studies varied; therefore, the conclusions of this review are preliminary. Research recommendations focus on promoting the growth of the evidence-base to support clinical practice.

Introduction

Phenylketonuria (PKU, OMIM 261600) is a rare genetic disorder with an incidence of approximately 1 in 10,000 (Donlon et al. 2004). Due to a deficiency in the enzyme phenylalanine hydroxylase, the amino acid phenylalanine (phe) cannot be sufficiently metabolised. PKU is primarily seen in a so-called 'classic' form in which the level of blood phe is above 1,200 μmol/L, as well in a milder variant, the prevalence of which is unknown, in which the blood phe level is between 600–1,200 μmol/L. In both cases, but to a necessarily greater degree in the case of classic PKU, phe builds up in the body, causing severe and irreversible cognitive impairment. However, this can be prevented to a considerable degree by a strict, lifelong, natural protein-restricted diet with amino acid supplements (see Koch et al. 2002). Although the aim of dietary treatment is to maintain blood phe concentrations within an acceptable target range, which is monitored via frequent blood samples, currently there is no universally accepted range, with different countries, and different clinics within countries, using varied management guidelines (Ahring et al. 2009; Feilliet et al. 2010).

Communicated by: BOLI-D-16-00290R3

Electronic supplementary material: The online version of this chapter (doi:10.1007/8904_2017_52) contains supplementary material, which is available to authorized users.

E. Medford · A. Wittkowski
School of Health Sciences, University of Manchester, Manchester, UK

E. Medford · A. Wittkowski (✉)
Greater Manchester Mental Health NHS Foundation Trust,
Manchester, UK
e-mail: anja.wittkowski@manchester.ac.uk

D.J. Hare
School of Psychology, Cardiff University, Cardiff, UK

Poor metabolic control in children and adolescents is associated with increased cognitive difficulties and poorer academic achievement (e.g., Azen et al. 1991; Chang et al. 2000). A meta-analysis of 40 studies by Waisbren et al. (2007) showed a 1.3–3.1 point reduction in Intelligence Quotient (IQ) for each 100 μmol/L increase in phe concentration. Furthermore, elevated phe levels have been associated with increased behavioural difficulties (Anjema et al. 2011; Smith and Knowles 2000) and poorer psychological wellbeing (Brumm et al. 2010; Clacy et al. 2014), with a hypothesised biological basis of these difficulties due to raised phe levels. Given the severe consequences of poor treatment adherence, it might be expected that very few children and adolescents have poor metabolic control. However, research indicates that this is not the case, with many children and adolescents having phe levels above the recommended range (Levy and Waisbren 1994; MacDonald et al. 2010, 2012; Walter et al. 2002; Walter and White 2004). For example, in a study with 330 patients, a quarter of 0–9 year-olds, half of 10–14 year-olds, and more than three-quarters of 15–19 year-olds had phe levels above their maximum recommended limits (Walter et al. 2002).

These issues can be considered within the broader context of treatment adherence in long-term treatments and/or chronic conditions (Horne et al. 2005; Haynes et al. 2008).

Despite the recognised difficulties with metabolic control, very few studies have examined interventions to improve treatment adherence, and those that have are limited and mainly uncontrolled (e.g., MacDonald et al. 2010). To inform interventions, it is necessary to identify the factors that affect treatment adherence for children and adolescents, and whether certain groups are at greater risk of poor metabolic control. A narrative review by MacDonald et al. (2010) highlighted a number of influences on dietary adherence, including patient age, social pressures, educational achievement of carers, and level of family cohesion [marital/cohabiting status of parents (Olsson et al. 2007)]. However, to date, there has been no systematic review of the factors affecting metabolic control for children and adolescents with PKU.

The aim of this review was to identify factors that were robustly linked with treatment adherence by examining studies reporting a statistical examination of the association between demographic and/or psychosocial factors relating to children and adolescents with PKU and their families, and metabolic control, as assessed by blood phe concentration.

Method

Search Strategy

A systematic search of Ovid Medline, PsychInfo, Embase, and EBSCO CINAHL was performed on 11th December 2015. Search terms were Phenylketonuria AND adheren* OR diet* OR treatment OR complian* OR control OR phenylalanine OR outcome* OR concordan*. Search limitations included English language, children and adolescents (0–18 years) and years 1985–2015.

Figure 1 presents an outline of the search process based on Preferred Reporting Items for Systematic Reviews and Meta-Analyses (PRISMA) guidelines (Moher et al. 2009). Studies were included if they (1) reported a statistical examination of the association between one or more demographic or psychosocial factor(s) and metabolic control (as measured by blood phe concentration) for children and adolescents with PKU, (2) were in the English language, and (3) were published in a peer-reviewed journal between 1985–2015. Case series and review papers were excluded.

Titles and abstracts were screened for inclusion by the first author and relevant abstracts were selected for full-text review ($n = 62$). Full text articles were assessed for eligibility and excluded if they did not meet the inclusion criteria. Any uncertainty about eligibility was resolved via discussion with another author. Six full text articles could not be accessed via inter-library loan, internet search, or by contacting authors via email. Twenty-eight papers were excluded: 16 did not examine the association between one or more demographic or psychosocial factor(s) and metabolic control and 12 reported a relationship but did not examine the association(s) statistically. Reference lists of included papers were manually examined, yielding one additional paper; thus, 29 studies were included. Data were extracted and entered into a database by the first author (see Supplementary Table 1).

Quality Assessment

The Quality Assessment Tool for Studies with Diverse Designs (QATSDD) was used to assess study quality (Sirriyeh et al. 2012). The QATSDD has shown good reliability and validity and was chosen due to the diverse methodologies of the included studies.

The 14 QATSDD items relating to quantitative studies were rated on a 4-point scale from 'not at all' (0) to 'complete' (3). The item scores were summed to provide a

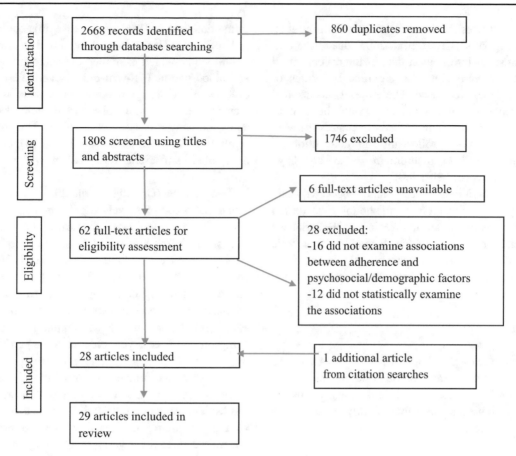

Fig. 1 Flowchart demonstrating literature-review procedure

total score, with a maximum score of 42 (see Supplementary Table 2). The first author rated all studies, and another author independently rated five studies (17%) to determine inter-rater reliability, which was good ($\kappa = 0.71$).

Results

Twenty-nine studies were included in this review, representing 1,784 participants with PKU (including children, adolescents and adults, see Supplementary Table 1 for participant age ranges). Sample sizes ranged from 13 to 167 participants and the sample characteristics that were reported varied greatly. Most studies provided information on patient age and sex, but few provided further details, such as socioeconomic status and ethnicity, alongside country of completion, with the most common country being the USA ($n = 11$). Of the 29 studies, 19 were cross-sectional, 7 were longitudinal, and 3 were intervention studies. Two of the intervention studies were pre-post designs with no control group (Gleason et al. 1992; Singh et al. 2000), and one was a randomised controlled trial (Durham-Shearer et al. 2008), with participants allocated to the intervention (educational resource) or control group (no

educational resource). Whilst all studies statistically examined associations between demographic or psychosocial factors and blood phe levels, many studies ($n = 13$) did not have this as their primary objective.

Quality Ratings

Quality ratings ranged from 14 to 34 (% of maximum score range 33–81%), with a mean of 26 (61%). Reasons for low ratings included having weak references to theory, limited rationale for choice of data collection tools, limited assessment of the reliability and validity of measurement tools, minimal evidence of user involvement in design, and minimal discussion of study limitations. Several studies also had small sample sizes, very few provided evidence that the sample size was considered in terms of analysis, and some did not provide a clear rationale for choice of analytic method. Only one study (Hood et al. 2014) provided separate effect sizes for significant findings and further inspection of the reported results identified that some post-hoc effect sizes could be computed for significant findings in five studies (Fehrenbach and Peterson 1989; Gleason et al. 1992; Arnold et al. 1998; Weglage et al. 1999; Griffiths et al. 2000) but that this was not

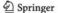

possible for four studies (Verkerk et al. 1994; Griffiths et al. 2000; Singh et al. 2000; Crone et al. 2005) due to the lack of relevant statistical information data in the papers. In all other cases, there were either no significant findings or correlational analyses were used. Therefore, it was decided that a comprehensive meta-analysis would be neither appropriate nor feasible and individual effect sizes (d) were reported where possible, following the convention of reporting small ($d = 0.2$), medium ($d = 0.5$) and large ($d = 0.8$) effect sizes (Cohen 1988).

Finally, on observation, an association between study quality and year of publication or methodological design was not evident. As this is the first review of the influence of psychosocial and demographic factors on metabolic control for children and adolescents, all studies were retained to provide a comprehensive overview of the available research.

Study Findings

Studies were grouped according to whether they examined the influence of child, parent or other family factors on metabolic control: 24 assessed child factors, 14 parent factors, and 8 reported on other family factors (see Supplementary Table 3).

Child Factors

Of 16 studies that examined the association between child age and metabolic control, 7 used correlational analyses, with 6 reporting a positive correlation (Al-Qadreh et al. 1998; Freehauf et al. 2013; McMurry et al. 1992; Schulz and Bremer 1995; VanZutphen et al. 2007; Vilaseca et al. 2010), and 1 reported no significant correlation (Arnold et al. 1998). Five Pearson's r coefficients ranged from 0.35–0.64, and one Spearman's rho coefficient was 0.62 (Freehauf et al. 2013). However, the positive correlation reported by Vilaseca et al. (2010); Pearson's $r = 0.63$ might be partially explained by an increase in target blood phe level for 6–12 year-olds (<600 µmol/L) compared to under 6-year-olds (<480 µmol/L). An additional study (Crone et al. 2005) found a quadratic rather than linear association between age and metabolic control, with blood phe increasing after 13 years.

One study (Freehauf et al. 2013) found a positive correlation between age and blood phe for over 12-year-olds (Spearman's rho $= 0.48$), but not for under 12-year-olds. When using a measure of difference score between phe level and target level, a significant correlation remained with age for over 12-year-olds (Spearman's rho $= 0.48$), indicating a progressive reduction of metabolic control

from adolescence. If this is the case, this could explain the lack of a significant correlation found in Arnold et al.'s (1998) study, which examined the association between age and blood phe in 1–8-year-olds. Nevertheless, in a sample of 8–19-year-olds, age was not significantly associated with metabolic control when phe was dichotomised into poor and good control (Olsson et al. 2007). However, as only a small proportion had poor control ($n = 14$), there might not have been sufficient statistical power to identify an association.

Two studies (Griffiths et al. 2000; Viau et al. 2011) found that blood phe levels significantly increased year-by-year with age, and eight studies found that blood phe was significantly higher for those above 6 years of age (Gokmen-Ozel et al. 2008; Vilaseca et al. 2010), 8 years (Al-Qadreh et al. 1998), 10 years (Hood et al. 2014), 12 years (McMurry et al. 1992; Vilaseca et al. 2010), and 14 years (Weglage et al. 1999). However, in Gokmen-Ozel et al.' (2008) study, the increase in phe for over 6-year-olds compared to under 6-year-olds might be partially explained by an increase in target phe levels from age 6.

Two studies examined the proportion of children who achieved good metabolic control and found contrasting results: Vilaseca et al. (2010) discovered that the proportion with good control decreased with increasing age (from under 6 years, to 6–12 years, to over 12 years), but Hartnett et al. (2013) found no significant difference between under 6 and 6–12-year-olds, whilst Cotugno et al. (2011) observed that more over 10-year-olds achieved target phe levels than under 10-year-olds, apparently contradicting studies showing reduced metabolic control with age.

Three studies (Hartnett et al. 2013; Hood et al. 2014; Viau et al. 2011) examined the relationship between age and variability in phe levels, but their findings showed no significant associations.

Sex

There was no significant relationship with blood phe levels (Al-Qadreh et al. 1998; Freehauf et al. 2013; Vilaseca et al. 2010) and the proportion achieving target levels (Cotugno et al. 2011) did not significantly differ between male and female children, and sex did not predict phe levels (Olsson et al. 2007; Verkerk et al. 1994). Olsson et al. (2007) noted that sex had a borderline statistical significance in a subgroup of children whose parents had not separated, with a tendency toward lower phe levels in female children. In addition, in a sample of 6–17-year olds, the proportion with 70% or more of their phe levels within target range was significantly higher for females than males (MacDonald et al. 2011).

Child Knowledge

Three studies evaluated the impact of adolescent treatment programmes designed to improve treatment adherence (Durham-Shearer et al. 2008; Gleason et al. 1992; Singh et al. 2000). Gleason et al. (1992) identified that post-intervention improvements in knowledge were accompanied by reductions in blood phe level; however, other treatment factors, including motivational techniques, might have led to reduced levels rather than improved knowledge. Two studies (Durham-Shearer et al. 2008; Singh et al. 2000) reported that post-intervention improvements in PKU knowledge were not accompanied by sustained reductions in blood phe. However, the intervention studies were limited by small sample sizes (n ranged from 16–32), and did not examine the direct association between PKU knowledge and metabolic control. An additional study (Bekhof et al. 2003) found that knowledge of PKU did not significantly predict blood phe levels.

Other Child Factors

In their examination of the association between metabolic control and child attributional style, Antshel et al. (2004) measured using locus of control ratings for vignettes describing a young person with behavioural dysregulation or academic difficulties. Locus of control ratings were significantly correlated with blood phe level (Pearson's $r = 0.61$ for behavioural dysregulation vignettes and 0.43 for academic difficulties vignettes), with higher blood phe associated with a higher external locus of control. They suggested that children with a higher internal locus of control assumed more personal responsibility for treatment adherence, resulting in better metabolic control, or that children with a higher external locus of control felt more powerless over their condition, leading to reduced treatment adherence.

In their intervention study examining the associations between metabolic control, attitudes, and health beliefs relating to PKU, Singh et al. (2000) found that post-intervention improvements in attitudes and health beliefs (assessed by questionnaires based on previous research) were not accompanied by sustained reductions in blood phe levels.

Finally, Ievers-Landis et al. (2005) examined the associations between adherence strategies, perceived strategy effectiveness, perceived problem frequency and difficulty (assessed by semi-structured interview and Likert scales), and metabolic control. Higher child perceived strategy effectiveness was associated with lower blood phe levels (Pearson's $r = -0.68$), but perceived problem frequency and difficulty were not significantly associated with blood phe levels. In addition, children who used strategies coded as maladaptive for treatment adherence (e.g., avoiding problems) had higher blood phe levels than those who did not use maladaptive strategies.

Parent Factors

Three studies examined the association between parent income and metabolic control. Whilst Griffiths et al. (2000) found that chief earner income was positively correlated with blood phe, two other studies (MacDonald et al. 2008; Reber et al. 1987) failed to identify a significant correlation between metabolic control and income. Of the three studies examining the association between parent employment or occupational status and metabolic control, only Alaei et al. (2011) noted that children with employed parents had significantly lower blood phe levels than children with unemployed parents. Employment status was not significantly associated with metabolic control in MacDonald et al.'s (2008) study and occupational level did not predict blood phe in Verkerk et al.'s (1994) study.

Five studies examined the association between parents' educational level and metabolic control. According to Reber et al. (1987) and MacDonald et al. (2008), blood phe was not significantly associated with parents' level of education. Alaei et al. (2011) found that metabolic control was not significantly different for parents with different educational levels. Although Olsson et al. (2007) noted that parental educational level did not predict phe levels dichotomised into good and poor control, Shulman et al. (1991) identified that children's concurrent phe level was correlated with maternal (Pearson's $r = -0.27$) and paternal education ($r = -0.28$), with higher education associated with lower blood phe.

Three studies examined the association between parent knowledge of PKU (using questionnaires based on previous research) and metabolic control. Whilst Gokmen-Ozel et al. (2008) found a significant negative correlation between maternal exchange knowledge score and blood phe level (Pearson's $r = -0.17$), total knowledge scores were not significantly associated with metabolic control. Similarly, MacDonald et al. (2008) reported that mother's total knowledge of PKU was not associated with phe level, nor was their ability to calculate exchanges or estimate the number of phe exchanges in food portions. Although Bekhof et al. (2003) noted that higher parent knowledge predicted lower blood phe levels, this association disappeared when other confounders were adjusted for (pretreatment phe, dietary phe tolerance, parent age, parent educational level, and ethnicity).

Fehrenbach and Peterson (1989) examined the associations between parent problem-solving skills, parenting strategies, and metabolic control. Children with good metabolic control had parents who produced a higher number and higher quality of verbal responses to PKU problem scenarios than children with poor metabolic control. Furthermore, those with good metabolic control had families that were organised in a more hierarchical manner with more firmly fixed rules. However, Ievers-Landis et al. (2005) observed that parents using strategies coded as "authoritarian" had children with higher phe levels than those who did not. In addition, higher parent perceived strategy effectiveness was associated with lower phe levels (Pearson's $r = -0.64$), and higher ratings of problem frequency ($r = 0.55$), problem difficulty ($r = 0.79$) and affective intensity ($r = 0.61$) were associated with higher phe levels.

Crone et al. (2005) examined the associations between parent attitudes, subjective norms, self-efficacy and metabolic control. Children's blood phe levels were lower when parents' experiences were that their child adhered well to the diet, even if their phe levels were sometimes too high (attitudes), and when parents answered that having their child eat the synthetic protein substitute was easy (self-efficacy). However, blood phe levels were higher when parents answered that their relatives did not agree when their child deviated from the diet (subjective norm).

Antshel et al. (2004) examined the association between metabolic control and parent attributional style. The latter was explored by asking parents to rate their perceived 'locus of control' (Rotter 1966) (i.e. the degree to which a person perceives events to be under their own control [internal locus of control] or under the control of other people or events [external locus of control]) in a series of written vignettes describing a young person with PKU presenting with behavioural dysregulation or academic difficulties. The subsequent locus of control ratings was significantly correlated with blood phe level (Pearson's $r = 0.69$ for behavioural dysregulation vignettes and 0.52 for academic difficulties vignettes), with higher blood phe associated with a higher external locus of control. Antshel and colleagues suggested that parents with a higher external locus of control felt more powerless in relation to their child's condition, leading to reduced efforts in supporting treatment adherence.

Finally, two studies examined the relationship between parental distress and metabolic control, and found that parental distress, parenting-related stress, and marital satisfaction were not significantly associated with phe levels (Reber et al. 1987), and level of external stress was not significantly different for those with good and poor control (Fehrenbach and Peterson 1989).

Other Demographic Factors

Two studies from the Netherlands examined the association between parental country of origin and metabolic control (Crone et al. 2005; Verkerk et al. 1994). Children with parents who had emigrated from a different country had higher blood phe levels than children with Dutch parents, possibly because of barriers to accessing health care services for some immigrants, such as language difficulties. In their study of the relationship between parent age and metabolic control, MacDonald et al. (2008) found no significant association.

Other Family Factors

Four studies examined the associations between family composition factors and metabolic control. Children with separated or divorced parents were more likely to have higher phe levels than children with married or cohabitant parents (Alaei et al. 2011; Olsson et al. 2007), but family size/number of children was not associated with metabolic control (Alaei et al. 2011; MacDonald et al. 2008). Whilst Alaei et al. (2011) found that blood phe was positively correlated with the number of children with PKU (strength of correlation not reported), Crone et al. (2005) noted that the number of children with PKU did not predict phe level. Three older studies specifically examined the association between family cohesion [i.e. marital/cohabiting status of parents] and metabolic control using parent questionnaires. Two studies used the Family Adaptability and Cohesion Evaluation Scale (Reber et al. 1987; Shulman et al. 1991) and one used the Family Environment Scale (Fehrenbach and Peterson 1989). Although Shulman et al. (1991) reported that lower blood phe level was moderately associated with higher paternal and maternal family cohesion scores (Pearson's $r = -0.34$; -0.36, respectively), Reber et al. (1987) and Fehrenbach and Peterson (1989) found no significant association with metabolic control. Finally, Freehauf et al. (2013) found no significant association between distance from home to clinic and metabolic control.

Discussion

This systematic review examined 29 identified studies reporting a statistical examination of the association between one or more demographic or psychosocial factor(s) and metabolic control (as measured by blood phe concentration) for children and adolescents with PKU. Only studies reporting statistical analyses were included in order to identify the factors most robustly linked with metabolic control and the QATSDD was found to be a valid tool for assessing the methodological quality of the studies included in the current review. In summary, the included studies examined a range of child, parent and family factors and indicated some strong associations with blood phe levels. However, there were some areas of investigation with a paucity of studies, highlighting a need for further research in this area.

This review suggests that the most reproducible factor associated with blood phe level currently is child age. Sixteen studies examined child age, with the majority finding a progressive reduction in metabolic control with age, and some suggesting that this occurred from adolescence. Reported correlations between age and metabolic control ranged from 0.35–0.64, indicating moderate to large associations. A similar influence of age has been found in children with diabetes (Neylon et al. 2013), implying that this association may be common in other metabolic disorders. With increasing age, it is likely that increased independency from the family and heightened social pressures, for example, around food and lifestyle, contribute to reduced dietary adherence (Levy and Waisbren 1994). It was noted that all 16 studies reporting an association with age did not examine this as their primary aim, suggesting that demographic data are frequently examined in health-related studies as a secondary objective.

Following age, the next most reproducible factor was child sex, with six studies indicating no association with sex and one study finding that more females had 70% or more of their phe levels within target range than males (MacDonald et al. 2011). In this study, the endpoint measure of 70% or more levels within target range might have allowed greater sensitivity with regard to identifying more subtle differences in metabolic control between males and females.

Due to the small numbers of studies examining other child, parent, and family factors, it is difficult to draw firm conclusions regarding their influence. However, regarding child factors, the available research indicated that blood phe level was not associated with child knowledge of PKU, attitudes, health beliefs, perceived problem frequency, or perceived problem difficulty. Conversely, blood phe level showed moderate to large correlations with child attributional style, a strong correlation with perceived strategy effectiveness, and was significantly different for those using maladaptive and non-maladaptive strategies.

Regarding parent and family factors, the available findings indicated that metabolic control was associated with parenting strategies, attitudes, subjective norms, self-efficacy, perceived strategy effectiveness, perceived problem frequency, perceived problem difficulty, attributional style, affective intensity of problems, country of origin, and marital status. Conversely, metabolic control was not associated with or inconsistently associated with parent knowledge of PKU, parent age, parent distress, family size, number of children with PKU in the family, family cohesion, geographic proximity to clinic, and socioeconomic factors, such as parent income, education, and occupation. The inconsistencies in findings between studies could be a result of different study methodologies, measures and cohort characteristics. For example, in relation to socioeconomic factors, participants from different countries may experience different levels of social inequality, and therefore factors such as unemployment may have a greater impact on treatment adherence and availability of low protein foods and food substitutes in some countries than others.

Limitations

Whilst this review identified a number of factors related to metabolic control, it was difficult to draw firm conclusions due to both a paucity of studies in some areas of investigation and some inconsistent findings. Furthermore, the strength of conclusions that can be drawn is limited by the varied quality of the included studies. As highlighted by the QATSDD ratings, a number of studies had small sample sizes with no evidence of consideration of the sample size in terms of analysis, meaning that the power of some studies could have been limited. However, it should be noted that the potential recruitment pool of young people with PKU is small due to the rarity of the condition, and hence small sample sizes are common. Nevertheless, as studies often provided scarce sample descriptions and the majority used cross-sectional methodology, it is difficult to draw conclusions about cause and effect influences on metabolic control. Finally, as there was limited availability of articles during the search process (six full-text articles were not available), it is unknown whether these would have met the inclusion criteria and contributed to the results and conclusions of this review.

Recommendations for Clinical Practice

This review indicates that certain groups of young people may be at higher risk of poor treatment adherence, particularly older children and adolescents. It is therefore important that clinicians and parents are aware of the tendency for worsening metabolic control with age and consider providing extra support to older children (around age 12 and above). Whilst PKU clinics routinely provide information about PKU and associated dietary treatment to young people and their carers, this review indicated that child knowledge of PKU was not associated with metabolic control, and parental knowledge was only weakly or inconsistently associated. Thus, treatment knowledge is necessary but not sufficient for dietary adherence. To date, there are no effective interventions to improve treatment adherence in PKU but current management guidelines for PKU in the UK (NSPKU 2014) recommend that services should be multi-disciplinary with a clinical psychologist to focus on, among other things, promoting 'patient and parent motivation to comply with treatment'. On the basis of the current review, such work could usefully focus on child and parent attributional style, attitudes and self-efficacy.

Recommendations for Future Research

This review highlights that there is a paucity of studies examining the potential demographic or psychosocial influences on metabolic control for young people with PKU, which appears to be in contrast to other metabolic conditions, such as diabetes, where metabolic control has been associated with factors such as ethnicity, personality characteristics and coping style (Neylon et al. 2013). Whilst currently unexplored, it is possible that these factors also influence treatment adherence for children with PKU. One of the reasons for limited research in this field is the small sampling pool due to the rarity of the condition, which makes it difficult to recruit sufficient numbers of patients. It is therefore recommended that future studies promote increased recruitment by working more in partnership with clinicians, patients, carers and support groups (DeWard et al. 2014).

It is important that future studies provide more information about participant characteristics, such as socioeconomic details, particularly as these may impact treatment adherence outcomes. In addition, more longitudinal studies are needed to help ascertain cause and effect influences on metabolic control and to explore whether other variables mediate the associations between factors such as age and metabolic control, such as increased social pressures. Although this is currently an emerging evidence-base, further studies could design and examine interventions to improve treatment adherence, informed by the factors highlighted in this review.

A further area for future research would be to examine treatment adherence from a health economics perspective and incorporate cost-benefit analyses alongside psychological and physiological data.

It is also important to acknowledge that small sample size is likely to continue to be an issue in future research in this field (Griggs et al. 2009). Therefore, further research could be informed by recent methodological thinking, for example, Abrahamyan et al.'s (2014) toolkit for conducting clinical trials with rare disorders and proposals to incorporate Bayesian statistical techniques into such studies (Billingham et al. 2001).

Conclusion

This review was the first to systematically examine studies reporting a statistical examination of the association between demographic or psychosocial factors and metabolic control for children and adolescents with PKU. Findings suggested that the most reproducible association was with child age, with control worsening with increasing age. Whilst a number of other factors were associated with blood phe levels, the evidence-base was small with some methodological limitations, and therefore the conclusions of this review are preliminary. This review highlights a paucity of research examining many demographic or psychosocial influences on metabolic control for young people with PKU. Research recommendations are therefore targeted towards promoting the growth of the evidence-base to support clinical practice.

Acknowledgements   We would like to express our sincere gratitude to Katie Carpenter for her assistance with this literature review.

Synopsis

This systematic review identified that whilst a range of demographic and psychosocial variables were associated with metabolic control for children with phenylketonuria, the most reproducible association was with child age.

Compliance with Ethics Guidelines

Conflict of Interest

Emma Medford, Dougal Hare and Anja Wittkowski declare that they have no conflicts of interest.

Informed Consent

All procedures followed were in accordance with the ethical standards of the responsible committee on human experimentation (institutional and national) and with the Helsinki Declaration of 1975, revised in 2013. However, as this article does not contain any studies with human or animal subjects performed by any of the authors, informed consent was not required.

Details of the Contributions of Individual Authors

Emma Medford contributed to identifying the review question, planning the search process and reporting, carrying out all aspects of the method section, and writing the majority of the article.

Dougal Hare contributed to identifying the review question, analysing and interpreting the results and to finalising this article.

Anja Wittkowski contributed to identifying the review question, planning the search process and reporting, screening articles, and finalising this article.

References

Abrahamyan L, Diamond IR, Johnson SR, Feldman BM (2014) A new toolkit for conducting clinical trials in rare disorders. J Popul Ther Clin Pharmacol 21(1):e66–e78

Ahring K, Bélanger-Quintana A, Dokoupil K et al (2009) Dietary management practices in phenylketonuria across European Centres. Clin Nutr 28:231–236

Alaei M, Asadzadeh-Totonchi G, Gachkar L, Farivar S (2011) Family social status and dietary adherence of patients with phenylketonuria. Iran J Pediatr 21:379–384

Al-Qadreh A, Schulpis KH, Athanasopoulou H et al (1998) Bone mineral status in children with phenylketonuria under treatment. Acta Paediatr 87:1162–1166

Anjema K, van Rijn M, Verkerk PH et al (2011) PKU: high plasma phenylalanine concentrations are associated with increased prevalence of mood swings. Mol Genet Metab 104:231–234

Antshel KM, Brewster S, Waisbren SE (2004) Child and parent attributions in chronic pediatric conditions: phenylketonuria (PKU) as an exemplar. J Child Psychol Psychiatry 45:622–630

Arnold GL, Kramer BM, Kirby RS et al (1998) Factors affecting cognitive, motor, behavioral and executive functioning in children with phenylketonuria. Acta Paediatr 87:565–570

Azen CG, Koch R, Friedman EG et al (1991) Intellectual development in 12-year-old children treated for phenylketonuria. Am J Dis Child 145:35–39

Bekhof J, Van Spronsen FJ, Crone MR et al (2003) Influence of knowledge of the disease on metabolic control in phenylketonuria. Eur J Pediatr 162:440–442

Billingham L, Malottki K, Pritchard M, Steven N (2001) Trials in rare diseases: the need to think differently. Trials 12(Suppl 1):A107

Brumm VL, Bilder D, Waisbren SE (2010) Psychiatric symptoms and disorders in phenylketonuria. Mol Genet Metab 99:59–63

Chang PN, Gray RM, O'Brien LL (2000) Patterns of academic achievement among patients treated early with phenylketonuria. Eur J Pediatr 159:96–99

Clacy A, Sharman R, McGill J (2014) Depression, anxiety, and stress in young adults with phenylketonuria: associations with biochemistry. J Dev Behav Pediatr 35:388–391

Cohen J (1988) Statistical power analysis for the behavioral sciences, 2nd edn. Lawrence Erlbaum Associates, Hillsdale, NJ

Cotugno G, Nicolo R, Cappelletti S et al (2011) Adherence to diet and quality of life in patients with phenylketonuria. Acta Paediatr 100:1144–1149

Crone MR, Van Spronsen FJ, Oudshoorn K et al (2005) Behavioural factors related to metabolic control in patients with phenylketonuria. J Inherit Metab Dis 28:627–637

DeWard SJ, Wilson A, Bausell H et al (2014) Practical aspects of recruitment and retention in clinical trials of rare genetic diseases: the phenylketonuria (PKU) experience. J Gene Couns 23:20–28

Donlon J, Levy H, Scriver C (2004) Hyperphenylalaninemia: phenylalanine hydroxylase deficiency. In: Scriver BA, Beaudet AL, Sly WS, Valle D, Vogelstein B, Childs B (eds) The metabolic and molecular bases of inherited disease. McGraw-Hill, New York

Durham-Shearer SJ, Judd PA, Whelan K, Thomas JE (2008) Knowledge, compliance and serum phenylalanine concentrations in adolescents and adults with phenylketonuria and the effect of a patient-focused educational resource. J Hum Nutr Diet 21:474–485

Fehrenbach AM, Peterson L (1989) Parental problem-solving skills, stress, and dietary compliance in phenylketonuria. J Consult Clin Psychol 57:237–241

Feilliet F, van Spronsen FJ, MacDonald A et al (2010) Challenges and pitfalls in the management of phenylketonuria. Pediatrics 126:333–341

Freehauf C, Van Hove JL, Gao D, Bernstein L, Thomas JA (2013) Impact of geographic access to care on compliance and metabolic control in phenylketonuria. Mol Genet Metab 108:13–17

Gleason LA, Michals K, Matalon R, Langenberg P, Kamath S (1992) A treatment program for adolescents with phenylketonuria. Clin Pediatr 31:331–335

Gokmen-Ozel H, Kucukkasap T, Koksal G et al (2008) Does maternal knowledge impact blood phenylalanine concentration in Turkish children with phenylketonuria? J Inherit Metab Dis 31:S213–S217

Griffiths PV, Demellweek C, Fay N et al (2000) Wechsler subscale IQ and subtest profile in early treated phenylketonuria. Arch Dis Child 82:209–215

Griggs RC, Batshaw M, Dunkle M et al (2009) Clinical research for rare disease: opportunities, challenges, and solutions. Mol Genet Metab 96:20–26

Hartnett C, Salvarinova-Zivkovic R, Yap-Todos E et al (2013) Long-term outcomes of blood phenylalanine concentrations in children with classical phenylketonuria. Mol Genet Metab 108:255–258

Haynes RB, Ackloo E, Sahota N et al (2008) Interventions for enhancing medication adherence. Cochrane Database Syst Rev 2 (2):CD000011

Hood A, Grange DK, Christ SE et al (2014) Variability in phenylalanine control predicts IQ and executive abilities in children with phenylketonuria. Mol Genet Metab 111:445–451

Horne R, Weinman J, Barber N et al (2005) Concordance, adherence and compliance in medicine taking. Report for the National Co-ordinating Centre for NHS Service Delivery and Organisation R & D (NCCSDO). NCCSDO, London

Ievers-Landis CE, Hoff AL, Brez C et al (2005) Situational analysis of dietary challenges of the treatment regimen for children and adolescents with phenylketonuria and their primary caregivers. J Dev Behav Pediatr 26:186–193

Koch R, Burton B, Hoganson G, Peterson R et al (2002) Phenylketonuria in adulthood: a collaborative study. J Inherit Metab Dis 25:333–346

Levy HL, Waisbren SE (1994) PKU in adolescents: rationale and psychosocial factors in diet continuation. Acta Paediatr Suppl 407:92–97

MacDonald A, Davies P, Daly A et al (2008) Does maternal knowledge and parent education affect blood phenylalanine control in phenylketonuria? J Hum Nutr Diet 21:351–358

MacDonald A, Gokmen-Ozel H, van Rijn M, Burgard P (2010) The reality of dietary compliance in the management of phenylketonuria. J Inherit Metab Dis 33:665–670

MacDonald A, Nanuwa K, Parkes L et al (2011) Retrospective, observational data collection of the treatment of phenylketonuria in the UK, and associated clinical and health outcomes. Curr Med Res Opin 27:1211–1222

MacDonald A, van Rijn M, Feillet F et al (2012) Adherence issues in inherited metabolic disorders treated by low natural protein diets. Ann Nutr Metab 61:289–295

McMurry MP, Chan GM, Leonard CO, Ernst SL (1992) Bone mineral status in children with phenylketonuria – relationship to nutritional intake and phenylalanine control. Am J Clin Nutr 55:997–1004

Moher D, Liberati A, Tetzlaff J, Altman DG (2009) Preferred reporting items for systematic reviews and meta-analyses: the PRISMA statement. Ann Intern Med 151:264–269

Neylon OM, O'Connell MA, Skinner TC, Cameron FJ (2013) Demographic and personal factors associated with metabolic control and self-care in youth with type 1 diabetes: a systematic review. Diabetes Metab Res Rev 29:257–272

NSPKU (National Society for PKU) (2014) Management of phenylketonuria: a consensus document for the diagnosis and management of children, adolescents and adults with phenylketonuria (PKU). The National Society for Phenylketonuria (UK) Ltd, Purley

Olsson GM, Montgomery SM, Alm J (2007) Family conditions and dietary control in phenylketonuria. J Inherit Metab Dis 30:708–715

Reber M, Kazak AE, Himmelberg P (1987) Phenylalanine control and family functioning 48 in early-treated phenylketonuria. J Dev Behav Pediatr 8:311–317

Rotter JB (1966) Generalized expectancies for internal versus external control of reinforcement. Psychol Monogr 80:1–28

Schulz B, Bremer HJ (1995) Nutrient intake and food consumption of adolescents and young adults with phenylketonuria. Acta Paediatr 84:743–748

Shulman S, Fisch RO, Zempel CE et al (1991) Children with phenylketonuria: the interface of family and child functioning. J Dev Behav Pediatr 12:315–321

Singh RH, Kable JA, Guerrero NV et al (2000) Impact of a camp experience on phenylalanine levels, knowledge, attitudes, and health beliefs relevant to nutrition management of phenylketonuria in adolescent girls. J Am Diet Assoc 100:797–803

Sirriyeh R, Lawton R, Gardner P, Armitage G (2012) Reviewing studies with diverse designs: the development and evaluation of a new tool. J Eval Clin Pract 18:746–752

Smith I, Knowles J (2000) Behaviour in early treated phenylketonuria: a systematic review. Eur J Pediatr 159:89–93

VanZutphen K, Packman S et al (2007) Executive functioning in children and adolescents with phenylketonuria. Clin Genet 72:13–18

Verkerk PH, Van Spronsen FJ, Van Houten M et al (1994) Predictors of mean phenylalanine levels during the first five years of life in patients with phenylketonuria who were treated early. Acta Paediatr Suppl 83:70–72

Viau KS, Wengreen HJ, Ernst SL et al (2011) Correlation of age-specific phenylalanine levels with intellectual outcome in patients with phenylketonuria. J Inherit Metab Dis 34:963–971

Vilaseca MA, Lambruschini N, Gomez-Lopez L et al (2010) Quality of dietary control in phenylketonuric patients and its relationship with general intelligence. Nutr Hosp 25:60–66

Waisbren SE, Noel K, Fahrbach K, Levy H (2007) Phenylalanine blood levels and clinical outcomes in phenylketonuria: a systematic literature review and meta-analysis. Mol Genet Metab 92:63–70

Walter JH, White FJ (2004) Blood phenylalanine control in adolescents with phenylketonuria. Int J Adolesc Med Health 16:41–45

Walter JH, White FJ, Hall SK et al (2002) How practical are recommendations for dietary control in phenylketonuria? Lancet 360:55–57

Weglage J, Pietsch M, Denecke J et al (1999) Regression of neuropsychological deficits in early-treated phenylketonurics during adolescence. J Inherit Metab Dis 22:693–705

Printed in the United States
By Bookmasters